Keep Your Marbles
A field guide for defanging
our fears of cognitive decline

Cliff Arceneaux, MMS, PA-C

Dedication

This book is dedicated to my fantastic wife and kids
whose belief in me kept pushing this book along.
Without them and their support, there would be no book.
So, if this book helps you, thank them first.

Acknowledgments

I have been greatly influenced and helped over the years by the work of Dr T. Colin Campbell, Dr Caldwell Esselstyn, Dr John McDougall and the indefatigable Dr Michael Greger. I am grateful for their years of work and generosity with their time.

I also need to thank my editor, Rachael Garrity, for helping craft my ideas and for giving me much support and good vibes throughout this process.

I am also very grateful to my wife for her love, and her support. For her critical eye and ear and for listening to me whine over the years. Who knew writing a book can take so long?

A big thank you to my mom and dad.
They did an awesome job raising me, and I am grateful.

And a special thank you to my dad for never giving up, even during the multiple times
when it would have been so very easy
to do so.
It was, is and always will be inspiring.

Contents

Introduction

Grandpa Clay was the strongest man I knew when I was a kid. We knew this as fact, mostly because he always told us, but also because he loved to grab us and show off his strength. I have no idea how tall Grandpa was in real life, but to us, he was a giant with a barrel chest and a booming voice. An avid hunter, he filled any room he entered. I remember riding home in his truck from field trials, running rabbits in the woods with his beagles. He would drive 70 mph with both windows rolled down, zooming down the interstate, loudly singing over the noise. His bass voice drowned out everything else.

Grandpa never wanted to get old and sickly. Unfortunately, his plan to have a massive heart attack and die early failed miserably. If the news told him that so & so was bad for you, he would eat two of them. The arteries of his heart clogged, yes, but not enough for The Big One. The arteries in his brain also started to harden, causing some mild strokes and memory loss. I remember talking with him about it.

"I live in a happy world," he said. He couldn't remember anything long enough to worry about it. The fun part was that he forgot all the old grudges and resentments he had carried around for years. All he could remember was that he had strong feelings for That Guy, so he assumed they were great friends. He inadvertently reconciled with old enemies, much to the confusion of his kids.

"But Dad, you raised us to hate That Guy."

"I did not. We've been friends for years!"

In the end though, he was reduced to a shell of his former greatness. He became the sickly old man he had always feared he would become.

Dementia has claimed more than one victim in my family. If Grandpa was the strongest man I knew, Mom Walker was the sweetest woman. Loving and doting, she left me with warm and wonderful memories of my early childhood of her reading me my favorite book, *Peter & the Wolf*. Sadly, by the time I had grown up enough to start to really get to know my family as actual people, she was already Less Than and had started to fade. Like so many others, she required 24/7 care, and at the end of her life had lost everything.

My Aunt Naomi's symptoms started much earlier. She had been a hoarder, but even that activity was partly due to forgetting what she already had, as well as a way to deal with the anxiety that plagues so many people with memory problems.

I have to do something.

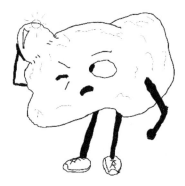

2020 was a memorable year in its own right. In the middle of the global pandemic and national riots, our little family was grappling with its own world-shaking problems.

My mother-in-law, Diane, had been diagnosed with dementia five years earlier. The good news for her brand of dementia was also the bad news. Once she was diagnosed, she declined fairly quickly. Diane had always been a wonderful, masterful chef, and was happy showing love to her friends and family through food. It hurt everyone when she could no longer bake even the simplest cake, or her internationally famous French Toast Logs. Holding a thought long enough to follow any recipe, even one of her own, became impossible.

My kids have good memories of sitting on the couch at our house with Diane, watching Andy Griffith reruns. They became really good at reminding Gammaw to sit back down, relax: "Everything is fine." It was one of the few ways we could give my father-in-law a break. My heart broke with the wrenching irony that it was my kids who were babysitting their grandmother, not the other way around. Christmas 2019, Diane experienced a significant decline, eventually landing in hospitals and rehabs (just before the COVID19 pandemic broke). She came home on Hospice in February, lasting only a few weeks. We are blessed to have had a wonderful, large funeral full of family and friends, one of the last in the country before the lockdown.

Frightfully soon afterward, my dad had a stroke. I was unable to go see him due to the travel restrictions. But he looked really bad on those first few Skype calls. His memory had been affected as well. He recovered well, but he is still aware that "I just forget stuff now."

At about that same time, one of the pillars in our local church started to have noticeable problems with her memory.

That's when it hit me: I have to do something. I have been working in medicine since 2000, having graduated from Wake Forest School of Medicine in 2006 as a physician assistant. I worked in geriatrics for eight years, grappling with dementia on a daily basis. I have spent the last three-to-four years digging through

3

books, journals, studies trying to find something, anything that would help. I knew what I had to do. I would write a book. The one you are currently reading.

This book represents a comprehensive expansion of a handout I have been giving my patients for years. I liked writing it out to the patients as we talked. That seemed more personal than just giving them a commercially produced handout. And it helped guide the discussion as to what was important. It was simply titled *The Memory Protocol* and incorporated a brief list of lifestyle interventions that had been proven to work in a variety of studies.

The Memory Protocol

1. Diet:
   Eat mostly plants, some meat
       (borrowed from Michael Pollan)
   Reduce sugar intake
   Avoid dairy

2. Exercise:
   At least 30 mins, just enough to get mildly sweaty, and get your heart rate up just a little bit. Walking is great. If you can do more, even better.

3. Sleep:
   Get around eight hours every night.
   Practice "sleep hygiene." (Caffeine is the enemy of sleep; no TV right before bed, etc.)

4. Deal with your stress:
   Do not avoid people; don't isolate yourself.
   Find/create more joy.
   Watch less TV; avoid cable news altogether.

The original idea behind this book was to take that simple list and add the kind of references and details that could help my patients and their families execute the plan we discussed. I saw it as a way to shed a ray of hope into their lives even during that first meeting when they have been crushed by the devastating diagnosis.

Each time those meetings take an hour, and even though my patients may feel like I've hit them with a firehose of information, we barely scratch the surface.

My hope for this book is to recreate for every reader the energy and hope we all feel at the end of those meetings. Yes, together we will be doing more than just scratching the surface, but I have been careful to avoid overwhelming those who read these pages with too much detail.

If you want the minute details, finish this book, and conscientiously follow this program for three to six months. At that point, your brain should be more than tuned up enough to tackle the heavy literature. There are plenty of journals, articles and books for those who want to geek out and dive into the weeds. And, for those of you who already have the constitution for it, enjoy the bibliography in the back of the book. You are welcome.

This book is written for anyone not interested in an exhaustive dive into pathophysiology of the various dementias, but who wants and needs hope. We will be discussing science-backed therapies with proven track records for arresting and sometimes even reversing memory loss.

What is not in the book? Magic potions and pills. There are no silver bullets for the fight against dementia. It has been called a "many-headed hydra." And rightly so, for it must be battled on numerous fronts. Like most all practitioners in this field, I have too many patients and families paying way too much money for really expensive supplements that at best do nothing and at worst make people sicker. I have a whole supplements section in the back of the book. But it's in the back of the book for a reason: pills and potions are supplemental to the meat and potatoes of the program. As wonderful as a tablet of turmeric is, it can't fix dementia. I know, I've tried it on folks. It's a nice piece to the puzzle, but quasi-useless by itself.

Similarly, we will not be discussing the latest commercially advertised product, or the latest Facebook rumor. If your Great Aunt Sally thinks eating ground up bee cartilage is making her feel better, great. More power to her. But I have not found any articles anywhere that have studied the effect of ground up bee cartilage on dementia, so we will not be discussing it here. (Yes, I actually looked.)

Dementia, a Primer

Alzheimer's and the various other forms of dementia are a scourge ravaging people across the globe. According to the Alzheimer's Association, there are 5 million people living with Alzheimer's in the US alone. A few other sobering statistics:

- Alzheimer's is the 5th leading cause of death in the US.

- One in three seniors in the US will die from one of the numerous types of dementia.

- Alzheimer's kills more people annually than breast cancer and prostate cancer combined.

- An estimated $305 billion was spent on care for Alzheimer's patients in 2020. That number is expected to balloon to $1.1 trillion in 30 years.

It's not hard for anyone to think of at least one friend or family member struggling with dementia, either directly as the patient, or indirectly as the caregiver.

Dementia or Alzheimer's

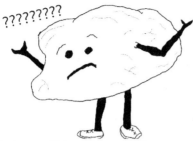

My first job in medicine was working as an acute care physical therapy tech at a hospital in Raleigh, NC. Which basically meant that among other glorious duties such as scrubbing out the hydrotherapy tanks for wound care, I caught people when they fell. If you or someone you know ever got out of bed in the hospital for therapy the day after their surgery and a concerned-looking person stood behind them as a human crash pad, that would have been me. A recurring part of the job was to go down to the ER to help patients learn how to properly use their new crutches. The most enjoyable part of these trips was the high number of patients, who probably thought of themselves as smart, educated people, who would exclaim, "I was so worried that I had broken my leg, but the doctor said it was only fractured!"

Now, I get a similar question regarding nomenclature. Unfortunately, it's nowhere near as funny: "Does Mom have Alzheimer's, or dementia?"

Webster's defines dementia as "a usually progressive condition (such as Alzheimer's disease) marked by the development of multiple cognitive deficits (such as memory impairment, aphasia, and the inability to plan and initiate complex behavior)." Dementia can be thought of as ice cream, and there are several types of memory loss flavors. So, Alzheimer's is a type of dementia. There are multiple flavors, and you really want to avoid all of them. Hence the reason for this book.

The different flavors or varieties of dementia point toward why it is so hard to treat. Both a quick search and an exhaustive dive into the research will give you pretty much the same answer: it's complicated. Numerous theories, lots of ideas, but little consensus. The most certain thing known right now is there is not one single cause for dementia. If there were, with all of the hours and money spent on research and treatment, it would have been found. No doubt we all would have stood around and thrown confetti at the ticker-tape parade down Main Street for the international heroes who found The Cure. Then we would all have stood in line for the shot or the pills to clean out the plaque in our brains. And as wonderful as that would be, the truth is there may be as many as 36 different factors that lead us to dementia.[1] *(Dale Bredesen, 2017.)*

There are research-backed clues that diet and lifestyle have a significant impact on brain health. For example, a randomized clinical trial released in 2011 put a group of men in their early 20s on a high fat, low carbohydrate diet. The men showed im-paired concentration, speed and mood after five days.[2] *(C. J. Holloway et al, 2011.)* A similar trial the same year showed that men placed on a high fat diet for seven days also suffered cognitive impairment.[3] *(Lindsay M. Edwards et al, 2011.)* The brilliantly titled review article from 2015, "Does the Brain Shrink as the Waist Expands?" looked at shrinkage within different portions of the brain across different ages as compared to the amount of fat the person carried. The conclusion: "Higher adiposity may be associated with frontal GM atrophy across all ages and parietal and temporal GM atrophy in middle and old age." Translation: As you get older, the fatter you are, the smaller brain you have.[4] *(Auriel. A. Willette et al, 2015.)*

Research also shows we can focus on the underlying cause of the worst offenders and start to heal the brain. And that is what our program—a simple, but powerful plan—does and you can start today. You might have to take a quick trip to the grocery store for supplies, but I will say again: you do not have to load up on tons of pills and potions or seek out gurus. In the back of the book there are a handful of supplements we have found to be helpful, but not so effective that you should put your faith solely in them. Not one pill, or four pills, not even 36 would be able to address all the factors that lead to the destruction and waste we refer to as "dementia."

Simply put: our research-based program relies on lifestyle changes to help heal the brain. Extremely powerful changes to your everyday routine can measurably affect your cognition, and at the same time reverse your heart disease and cure your diabetes. Our target list is a trio: Rust & Inflammation, Plumbing Problems, and Sugar Problems.

Inflammation & Rusting

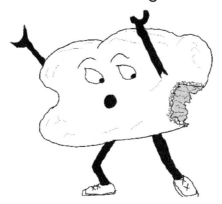

Why do we care about inflammation? Think about catching your little toe on the leg of the bed at night. Hurts, right? The toe feels like a bag of shattered glass doused with kerosene that ignites once you hit the bed, turns red and swells up. A red, angry, swollen toe is hard to bend, and hard to walk on. This is inflammation. Now, take that red swollen toe, and imagine it's your brain. An inflamed, unhappy brain does not work nearly so well as it is supposed to do. Caring about inflammation is important to brain health. Multiple studies of patients with dementia have found higher levels of inflammatory markers as compared to those without dementia. Anything we can do to lower the inflammation is going to be good for our hearts, brains, joints, lungs, you name it.[5] *(Luigi Ferrucci et al, 2018.)*

Chronic inflammation can lead to what is called "oxidative stress." To use some of your old SAT-test-taking skills, oxidative stress is to your brain what rust is to boats. It is actually the exact same chemical reaction. And just like you don't want to go to sea with a rusty boat, you don't want to go through life with a rusty brain.[6] *(Wen-Juan Huang et al, 2016.)*

Quick thought experiment: what happens when you cut up an apple and leave it on the table for five minutes? 15 minutes? An hour? It turns brown, gets mushy and tastes weird. This is because the oxygen in the air reacts with the enzymes in the apple. The oxygen molecules steal electrons from the apple's cells, wreaking havoc along the way and leading to a brown, mushy apple. Same thing happens with inflammation and your body. These rogue destabilized oxygen molecules fly through your body stealing electrons from other atoms until they're satisfied. Of course, this destabilizes the neighborhood, creating more rogue oxygen atoms (officially called "Reactive Oxygen Species"), which attack their neighbors who in turn attack their neighbors, much like your common zombie apocalypse. Zombie apocalypse movies can be entertaining on the screen, but not in your brain.

Plumbing Clogs

The amount of data linking atherosclerosis (hardening of the arteries) to dementia continues to build higher each day.[7] *(Limor Raz et al, 2016.)* Atherosclerotic lesions in the brain have been directly linked to Alzheimer's pathology. From blockages in the main arteries to even the microvascular areas, cerebrovascular lesions all work hand-in-hand with Alzheimer's pathology in almost every cell in your brain to make a huge mess.[8] *(Pedro M. Pimentel Coelho et al, 2012.)*

This effect even harkens back to Patient Zero, a nice lady named Auguste, who in 1904 was taken to Dr. Alzheimer in Frankfurt, Germany, for the now-familiar constellation of symptoms: anxiety, memory loss, "delusional." Dr. Alzheimer noted during her autopsy in 1907, "The larger cerebral vessels show arteriosclerotic change." [9] *(Alios Alzheimer et al, 1995.)*

By 1970, the idea of "cardiogenic dementia"[10]*(No authors listed, Lancet article, 1977.)* had started to gain traction. Cardiogenic dementia theory proposes that a brain deprived of oxygen due to constricted blood flow suffers greatly, even more so if that brain has a few miles on it. I explain to my patients that just like the heart, the brain has arteries all over it and in it. And again, just like the heart, those arteries can get blockages in them, constricting the blood flow to everything unfortunate enough to be trapped on the other side. And in both heart and brain, that is a very bad thing.

Autopsies on Alzheimer's patients have repeatedly found blockages in the central group of arteries called "The Circle of Willis," a superhighway deep in the brain that leads, among other places, to the memory centers.[11] *(Alex E. Roher et al, 2011.)* A 2016 autopsy study found that the more severe the blockages, the higher the odds of Alzheimer's disease, as well as of lower cognitive scores in general.[12] *(Zoe Arvanitakas et al, 2016.)*

OK, we know about dead brains, but what about the living? In 2014 researchers used CT angiography to measure the blockages in the brains of patients who had been diagnosed with early, mild cognitive impairment. After four years, the more severe the blockage in the arteries of the brain, the greater the patients' chances of developing full-blown Alzheimer's disease. Those with mild or stable blockages had a much greater chance of maintaining their cognitive functions. The researchers' conclusion? "An inefficient blood supply to the brain has very grave consequences on brain function."[13] *(Jie Zhu et al, 2014.)*

12

This relationship was further confirmed by a 2020 study analyzing the proteins associated with atherosclerosis. It found molecular links between cholesterol-fueled blockages in the arteries of the brain and dementia.[14] *(Aliza P. Wingo, et al, 2020.)* The relationship between vascular health and brain health is so strong, treatment of atherosclerosis and its root causes has been shown to slow the decline of Alzheimer's patients.[15] *(Yes Deschaintre et al, 2009.)*

Arteriosclerosis versus atherosclerosis? What's the difference?

It's easy to get lost in the medical lingo, especially when two terms that mean almost the same thing are excruciatingly similar, such as arteriosclerosis and atherosclerosis. They both refer to problems within the arteries and even end with the same tongue-twister.

Arteriosclerosis is the medical term for hardening of the arteries. Atherosclerosis is what we call it when arteries have been hardened due to an accumulation of plaque. Think about the ice cream analogy from before. Atherosclerosis is a flavor of arterio-sclerosis. Both should be avoided.

Sugar Problems

Slow, steady, progressive cognitive decline is yet another tragic side effect of diabetes mellitus at every age. Obviously, the older you are and the longer you have been diabetic, the worse your cognitive problems are likely to become. Terrifyingly enough, cognitive impairments can show up as early as age seven for Type 1 diabetics.[16] *(Geert Jan Bissels et al, 2018.)* A 2019 review article makes the case for "diabetes-related dementia," thought to be caused by a toxic soup of insulin resistance, inflammation, oxidative stress and AGEs (Advanced Glycation End products). AGEs are fats and proteins mutated into dangerous compounds after exposure to sugar. They are linked to increased vascular damage in diabetes, but also arthritis, heart disease and, you guessed it, dementia.[17] *(Alison Goldin et al, 2006.)* The good news is that researchers consider diabetes-related dementia to be reversible, because they have witnessed how improved glycemic control can in turn improve attention, focus and other symptoms.[18] *(Haruo Hanyu, 2019.)*

The reason for the link is not as clear as the link itself. Researchers have little doubt that multiple factors are in play, and one area of focus is insulin resistance. Insulin resistance has long been considered a driving force in diabetes, but now it is also becoming an area of much research and study as it pertains to dementia. Insulin resistance leads to higher and higher blood sugars, and then to more AGEs, inflammation and vascular damage. The brain itself can also become insulin resistant, directly affecting its ability to enjoy its preferred food source--glucose. As the brain becomes starved for food, it, well, starves. Treating the brain quasi-directly with intranasal insulin (squirted up into the nose rather than given as a shot in the belly) has been shown to help young diabetic males with cognition, but similar tests in geriatric diabetics were disappointing.[19] *(Steve E. Arnold, et al, 2018.)* Other researchers argue that brain injury and memory loss are caused not by the sugars being too high, but instead getting too low.[20] *(Graydon S. Meneilly, et al, 2016.)* Whatever the reason, it's clear being too sweet for too long is a terrible idea for brain health.

FAQ

Briefly, here are the most common questions I get from folks when we discuss dementia.

Genetics

There is a great deal of good science and of terrible fear swirling around Apolipoprotein E4 (ApoE4), better known as "The Alzheimer's Gene." According to the Alzheimer's Association, 40 to 65 percent of all Alzheimer's patients have the ApoE4 gene. If you have one set of the ApoE4 gene, your chance of developing Alzheimer's is much higher than normal. If you were given a matched set of the gene from your parents, your risk is depressingly high, but still not 100 percent. It's grim, but according to data produced by researchers at Loma Linda University, just using lifestyle changes such as the ones in this book can push back the development of symptoms 10 to 15 years even for a genetically pre-disposed person.[21] *(Dean and Ayesha Sherzai, 2017.)* In the case of my mother-in-law, instead of getting sick at 65 years of age, she would have been 80 years old. That's 15 extra years with the grand-kids. What a difference that would have made in all our lives.

Let's do some more math. If 40 to 65 percent of cases can be traced to the ApoE4 gene, that means that 35 to 60 percent of cases are due to. . .something else. And often that something else can be manipulated in our favor.

Ok, let's get back to ApoE4. You might be wondering what the point of having such a timebomb in our DNA is. Apolipoprotein E4 actually has to do with cholesterol transportation, but it is implicated in higher rates of inflammation and oxidative stress.[22] *(Laia Jofre-Monseny et al, 2008.)* Remember, short-term inflammation around an injury is a good thing. It rallies the defensive troops to fight any infections and get the repair crews in place and working. This is a good thing if you are walking barefoot hunting sabretooth tigers. It's a bad thing in today's world of proinflammatory foods and chronic stress.

Epigenetics is the study of how outside influences affect the way genes work in DNA. It's an interesting field that offers a great reason for hope for those with a strong family history of dementia, heart disease, diabetes, etc. You can influence your genes to create greater health, or crush disease.

If ApoE4 were the main cause of Alzheimer's, you would expect the rates of Alzheimer's to be the same across the world, right? You're born with the gene, you die with the disease, end of story. But the rates of Alzheimer's vary greatly, as much as ten-fold![23] (W.B. Grant, 1999.) If genetics were the main culprit, this would not be the case.

In 1996, researchers compared the prevalence of dementia in Japanese-American men, many of whom had immigrated to the US and were now living in Hawaii, eating a western diet of cheeseburgers and fast food to the rates of dementia of Japanese men living in Japan, eating a more traditional Eastern diet. Similar genetics, you would expect similar outcomes, right? Wrong. The Japanese-American men had higher rates of Alzheimer's than their genetic counterparts in Japan. In fact, despite their being from Japan, their risks were right in line with patients of European ancestry.[24] (L. White, et al, 1996.) Similar genes, different outcomes.

So, we should all move to Japan to save our brains? No, as Japan adopts the classic Western diet full of meat, sweets and high-fat dairy products, the country's rate of Alzheimer's disease climbs as well. In 1985, the rate of Alzheimer's was about 1 percent in Japan. As the population switched from sushi & green tea to cheeseburgers & milkshakes, the rate had climbed to 7 percent by 2008.[25] (W. B. Grant, 2016.) A study published in 2017 suggested the dementia rate had also risen to more than 15 percent by 2015.[26] (William Montgomery et al, 2017.) By 2020 a study had found equal rates of dementia among Japanese men and American men.[27] *(Yasuhiko Saito et al, 2020.)* Why? The genetic code for millions of Japanese men did not suddenly change over 20 years. How their genes reacted to their new diets and lifestyles I fear is what closed the gap. As more of the world eats the same foods and lives the same type of lifestyle, we should not be surprised when all our disease profiles start to look the same.

The fact that we can change our genetic destiny is wonderfully highlighted by the so-called "Nigerian Paradox."[28] *(Michael Greger et al 2015.)* Nigerians have the highest occurrence of the ApoE4 gene[29] *(B. Sepehrnia et al, 1989)* and yet the lowest rates of Alzheimer's disease![30] *(W. B. Grant, 1999.)* How is that possible? Nigerians have extremely low cholesterol levels thanks to a diet of mostly fruits, vegetables, grains, & legumes. And low cholesterol levels have been found to greatly reduce the chances of developing dementia, even in people with two copies of ApoE4![31] *(Mia Kivipelto et al, 2002)* These folks are able to "out eat" their genetics! This idea is at the heart of this book: there is hope, even if the odds appear to be stacked against you. You can fight back, and you can win.

Drugs

I always listen to patients and their families who tell me Such & Such drug "made me feel crazy/sleepy/stupid/confused." They are probably right.

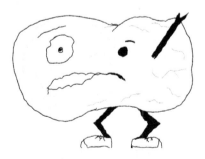

The American Geriatrics Society publishes "The Beers" list, highlighting what drugs are deemed inappropriate to be given to older patients.[32] *(No authors listed, 2019.)* The list is named after Dr. Beers, much like Angie's List (Now, Angi, I believe.) or Craigslist is named after, well, Angie and Craig. Updated every year, the Beers List contains a comprehensive set of medications people over the age of 65 should avoid. Not every drug on the list has been linked to cognitive impairment, but there are enough to give all of us pause.

For example, most of your older, commonly prescribed generic drugs for overactive bladder such as oxybutynin and tolterodine are linked to "confusion, hallucinations and sedation." Sometimes irreversible damage may be done. The class of medications known as "anticholinergics" is also strongly linked to an increased risk of dementia.[33] *(Carol A. C. Coupland et al, 2019.)* What is in the anticholinergic group? A household staple around the world, diphenhydramine is an over-the-counter drug used for allergy symptoms but also used in most over-the-counter sleep aids. Most Parkinson's drugs, as well as certain antidepressants and anti-psychotic drugs, are also linked.

If you or a member of your family might be affected, I highly suggest you take a look at the Beers list and talk with your primary health care practitioner about it.

Cliff's notes version of BEERS list. For full list and complete list of side effects, please reference the complete list at America Geriatrics Society web site.

Drug names & Family	Unwanted Side Effects
Antihistamines, both over the counter and by prescription, like Benadryl (diphenhydramine), Vistaril, Antivert, Phenergan, etc.	Risk of confusion, dry mouth, constipation headache, impaired memory, reduced cognitive function, behavioral disturbances, anxiety, and insomnia. Fights against most memory medications. Side effects worse when used as a sleep aid. Using diphenhydramine for treatment of severe allergic reaction still appropriate.
Certain antidepressants and antipsychotics such as Elavil, Anafranil, Norpramin, Pamelor, Paxil	Common instances of headache, impaired memory, reduced cognitive function, behavioral disturbances, anxiety, and insomnia. Increased risk of cerebrovascular accident (stroke) and greater rate of cognitive decline and death in persons with dementia.
Benzodiazepines such as Xanax Ativan, Restoril, Klonopin, Valium	All benzodiazepines increase risk of cognitive impairment, delirium, falls, fractures, and motor vehicle crashes in older adults.
Prescription sleep aids such as Lunesta, Ambien, etc.	Adverse events similar to those of benzodiazepines in older adults (e.g., delirium, falls, fractures); increased emergency department visits and hospitalizations; motor vehicle crashes
Muscle Relaxers such as Soma, Skelaxin, Robaxin, etc.	Most muscle relaxants poorly tolerated by older adults because of the adverse effects of headache, impaired memory, reduced cognitive function, behavioral disturbances, anxiety, and insomnia, sedation, increased risk of fractures; effectiveness at dosages tolerated by older adults questionable (i.e. all pain, no gain)
https://www.guidelinecentral.com/summaries/american-geriatrics-society-2015-updated-beers-criteria-for-potentially-inappropriate-medication-use-in-older-adults/#section-420	
The use of antipsychotics and antidepressants for behavioral problems of dementia or delirium can still be appropriate once nonpharmacological options (e.g., behavioral interventions) have failed or are not possible and the older adult is a threat to self or others.	

Surgery

It is well known that some people given anesthetics for major surgery don't always make it all the way back. I've seen many families come with similar stories: "Mom was fine; then she had [Surgery X], woke up confused and hasn't been the same since." One of the worst cases was a man who had several revisions of his joint replacement within a very short amount of time. In less than six months, the poor family watched helplessly as a fully functioning happy, grandpa became a lost, unhappy soul unable to feed or clean himself. A 2017 study of hip fracture patients found those who experienced delirium, had problems with blood pressure during or after surgery, were physically weak before surgery or all of the above were much more likely to develop new-onset dementia within a year after being released from the hospital.[34] *(Bjorn Erik Neerland et al, 2017.)* A meta-analysis published in 2020 confirmed delirium to be "significantly associated with long-term cognitive decline in both surgical and non-surgical patients."[35] *(Terry E. Goldberg et al, 2020.)*

The way I describe it to my patients is that the problem is not unlike Humpty Dumpty. The damage to the brain from any of the forms of dementia has been occurring for years. And then you get to a tipping point where the symptoms start to really accelerate. And the insult the body receives from major anesthesia, loss of blood pressure during surgery, and/or medications for pain or overactive bladder generates the push the brain needs to topple off the fence.

Again, dementia is multifactorial. No one thing has been found to be the sole cause. If it had, we could have cured this problem a long time ago. So, I don't blame a single surgery or even a drug regimen for causing Grandpa's dementia.

That being said, all of us want to do everything we can to preserve our beautiful brain tissue. Dig through the Beers list and the bottles in your cabinets and start throwing out anything that could contribute to future problems. And if you are having surgery, discuss with your anesthesiologist the most brain-healthy cocktail she or he can come up with.

Current state of treatment = pitiful

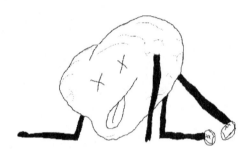

The FDA has approved only a handful of drugs to treat memory loss. Not one of them is cheap, and they all have extensive side effects. They are not a cure. Most of them at best slow down the symptoms of memory loss.

It is recommended that the main work-horse drug, donepezil, be started fairly early in the disease process to reduce the severity of a few symptoms for a time. Still, it does not slow down the rate at which the disease progresses. Donepezil and a sugar pill have about the same chance of assuring you will not end up needing a high level of care like a memory unit in a nursing facility. And the sugar pill has the exact same chance of preventing "adverse events or death" as the prescription pill.[36] *(C. Courtney et al, 2004.)*

A review of multiple studies of treating dementia with donepezil found "moderate evidence" that patients "experience small benefits in cognitive function, activities of daily living and clinician-rated global clinical state." It is important to remember, of course, that most studies only run 12 to 24 weeks, with only one small study looking at patients for one year. Higher doses might work better than lower doses, but the higher doses are associated with higher adverse effects, so patients usually stop the drug.[37] *(Jacqueline S. Birks et al, 2018)*

Aducanumab

In the summer of 2021, the FDA approved a new dementia drug, aducanumab, amidst much controversy. The first new drug approved in 18 years to treat Alzheimer's should have been met with praise and a ticker-tape parade, right? And it would have had the drug looked as if it actually worked.

Aducanumab is a monoclonal antibody infusion designed to target the amyloid plaques that form strangling tangles inside the brains of Alzheimer's patients. However, in 2019 the two Phase 3 trials for aducanumab were halted, because it appeared the drug was not helping the patients at all.

Later, the manufacturer ran the numbers again and found that while the first trial still showed no benefit whatsoever, the second trial did show a 22 percent decrease in the decline of the patients' cognition. Said another way, the rate at which the patients were getting worse slowed down by 22 percent. In terms of how it might look in the real world: "The clinical benefit amounted to about 3 months' worth of delay in decline over a year."[38] *(David S. Knopman et al, 2021.)* So as a group, the patients still declined, just a little slower maybe than the control group. The FDA was petitioned for approval. When the FDA's advisory panel took a hard look at the data, they ruled that a 22 percent decrease in the rate of decline over 18 months was not worth the significant side effects. Among the patients who received aducanumab, 41 percent experienced bleeding in and around the brain, severe headaches, confusion, delirium, falling and diarrhea, compared to 10 percent of the placebo patients who reported nothing more than getting a headache. While the panel was not unanimous, everybody voted no except for one hold-out who voted "uncertain." No one voted to approve this drug for the public.

In an unprecedented move, the FDA went against their own panel and approved the drug. Why? The FDA decided to concentrate on the fact that the drug reduced the amount of Amyloid Beta protein in the brain and ignored the fact that other trials of reducing amyloid plaques in the brain actually caused worse cognitive function and greater decline in daily living.[39] *(Michael F. Egan et al, 2019.)* Three of the members of the advisory panel loudly quit in protest.

Initially this once-a-month IV infusion that has close to a 50/50 chance of causing major brain bleeding was going to cost the patient $4,132 a month; $56,000 annually. For the cost of a brand new BMWx4, you could reduce the rate of decline in your mom's Alzheimer's by 22 percent in the first year. The manufacturer reduced the cost of aducanumab to $28,200 a year, presumably due to backlash over the cost and lack luster sales from all the negative publicity.[40] *(https://www.wsj.com/articles/biogen-cuts-price-for-alzheimers- drug-aduhelm-byhalf-11640001661.)*

Soon after this, the European version of the FDA decided not to approve aducanumab for use in the European Union. "Aducanumab does not appear to be effective at treating adults with early-stage symptoms," the European Medical Agency said, and may cause harm to Alzheimer's patients.[41] *((https://www.bbc.com/news/health-59699907.)*

The latest curve ball was Medicare's recently announcement the federal program would only pay for aducanumab for patients in certain approved clinical trials. [42] *(https:// www.statnews.com/ 2022/01/11/medicare-aduhelm-proposeddecision/)*

Aducanumab was originally approved only for patients with amyloid plaques that can be tracked by MRI and PET scans or lumbar punctures, and then only for patients who have very mild symptoms.

The Keep Your Marbles program is also for patients with very mild symptoms, but you don't have to spend more time and money on MRIs, and you certainly don't have to spend the cost of a new rather high-end car every single year to reap the benefits.

Only the strategies laid out in this book have been proven to stop or even reverse memory loss. That's why I am writing this book--to give people a chance. After nine long years treating dementia patients, I know pills are not the answer.

Are there any other new drugs on the horizon? Yes, plenty of hope-based contenders (roughly 125 at last count),[43] *(Elisabeth Mahase, 2021.)* some aiming at the exact same targets as the old drugs that don't work so well, so good luck with that. If they make it out of the research combine, those drugs focused on the same areas the KYM program targets, namely inflammation and/or the genetic expression of ApoE4, are likely to be heavily touted and also cost a fortune. Even practitioners in the field have no idea of potential side effects, other than a slimmer wallet, I am sure.

Don't get me wrong. I really hope they work, and I hope they work great. I hope they are game changers.

But I also know this KYM program already addresses inflammation and the gene expression of ApoE4. Why wait another five years to get help? Why wait at all? The whole point of this book is to get you started today, right now, without having to buy anything extra. Except maybe some broccoli.

Hope, lost and regained

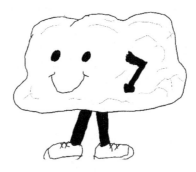

I was losing hope. I have had the great fortune of working in a variety of clinics in my career, from family medicine to cardiology to a prison infirmary. While I loved the relationships with my patients, and I truly felt it to be an honor to serve, I was losing hope. The pills I had been throwing at people were insufficient. And I didn't know any other way to treat anything. All through school we had been taught to let the patient go ahead and try diet and exercise, and when it fails put them on the pills. Because lifestyle interventions don't work, but the pills do.

But here's the problem: In cardiology people would dutifully take the handful of pills we gave to them, yet still have heart attacks and die. Some argue the quick heart attack deaths are preferable to slowly gasping out your last breaths in a hospital room, hoping your family can get there in time so you can say goodbye.

In geriatrics, I faced a similar problem. Our patients took at least one handful of pills a couple of times a day, and still got worse.

The visits I dreaded the most were the New Patient appointments, for which you walk in and see a whole family gathered around the patient. My heart would sink. You glance through the paperwork, see the below-average score on their memory screening test and respectfully listen to the family's heartbreaking story.

- "Mom is forgetting things, people, places. . . .She used to be so sharp. This isn't like her."

- "Dad is getting mean; he used to be so sweet."

- "My wife is seeing people in the house, talking to people who aren't there."

- "They found him wandering down the street, totally lost and confused."

We would start the standard workup: MRI of the brain to rule out tumors, strokes, etc.; use carotid ultrasounds to see if it were possible to open up blood flow; schedule a NeuroPsych consult to help pinpoint exactly where on the road the patient might be.

I got really good at explaining the decline, detailing what could be expected, holding their hands while I crushed any remaining hope of their family's ever being whole again.

Yes, there are pills, but they are expensive, have a lot of side effects and slow down the symptoms for anywhere from six months to two years at best.

No, the supplements advertised on TV don't work. I've already checked. Jellyfish don't get dementia, because jellyfish don't have brains, therefore the ground up jellyfish pills are not going to help.

After the appropriate wait, my colleagues and I would have the families come back to review the labs and MRI results, before discussing the right time to take the keys away, when to disconnect the stove and how long the average patient can go without needing 24/7 supervision. Trying to keep the patients as close to being themselves as we could, we would prescribe one memory pill at the start, then two, then add something else for depression.

Growing weary, I started to look around for anything else. Pills, potions, voodoo, whatever might work. Out of all the different protocols out there, common things began to emerge. Over and over again, lifestyle interventions worked so much better than the prescription pills. Some supplements seemed to be ok, but honestly just having folks eat their vegetables, get a good night's sleep and take a walk consistently improved the lives of patients.

From that research, I started my guinea pig groups.

I changed my pitch on the new-patient visits and started to present what would eventually be this book. I was very honest with the patients and their families. I presented two options: we can go traditional or experimental. The known pitfalls of the traditional approach: in the long term nothing we do is really going to make any difference. The experimental approach? The main problem again is that it might not work. But what if it did? Even if lifestyle intervention could only slow down the disease for a few years before we started the pills, we would consider that a win. These folks would be my guinea pig group. It worked on paper for others; we would see if it worked here in our clinic. Some families were polite, some were hostile, but some grabbed onto this information like it was a life preserver. Here is one of my favorite stories.

⬜ Poster Boy ⬜

An older gentleman who reminded me of a Dick Tracy villain, but in a good way, came to us with a diagnosis of Alzheimer's from a doctor he had been seeing. His wonderful, yet beleaguered, wife had grown weary with providers' throwing an ever-increasing pile of pills at her husband. The couple had once traveled extensively, but now being in unfamiliar places made him nervous. His broken mind could no longer deal with the stresses of travel; it was just too much to handle. He would start to hallucinate, get extremely anxious and basically suck all the fun out of any vacation. We reduced some of his medications, on the condition that they would replace the prescription regimen with The Memory Protocol. They were the first couple to really try it, and it worked. He quit getting worse. Not only quit getting worse--he improved!

Now, he was not "fixed" in the conventional or infomercial sense. His brain had been damaged quite a bit, so we went in knowing he wasn't going to magically turn 30 years old again. Sure, they still had their daily struggles, their good days, ok days and bad days. But he could travel and take up some of his hobbies again. They did not do the whole program 100 percent perfectly either. They only needed to do enough to start allowing the brain to heal. How much is enough? That varies from patient to patient, situation to situation.

Sadly, eventually his disease still progressed. The damage from before was too much to overcome. As he got worse, the protocol became harder to do, which meant it was followed less and less and he declined faster and faster. But we had snatched back a few good years for them, and for that we were grateful.

He was one of my first guinea pig patients, and he proved to me that we really were onto something.

Body of evidence

I like to talk to patients about *The Blue Zones*. Originally a study from National Geographic made into a book and now a book series and city planning movement, this work focuses on areas of the world where people live not only long, but well while they do it. Featured are places like Okinawa, Japan and Sardinia, Italy. And by long, I don't mean they can still play shuffleboard when they are 71 years old. I mean they can still beat you at shuffleboard at 101.
There are numerous things that the people living in five different places identified as Blue Zones have in common that are believed to contribute to their long lives: daily activity, daily time spent with

friends and family, plant heavy diets, sense of purpose, etc. I do not have the space in this book to go over everything covered in those books. I do encourage you to read them, though. I do highlight the movement and eating sections with my patients when we talk about brain health.

One of the Blue Zones is right here in the good ole U.S. of A. Loma Linda, California, is home to Loma Linda University and has a large population of Seventh Day Adventists. As part of their faith, Seventh Day Adventists take regular exercise and adhere to a plant-heavy diet. Some are pescatarians, most are some level of vegetarian, and some are full vegans. Studies of the church's members are excellent, because you can use them to compare these folks to their non-Adventist neighbors right down the street.

The Adventist health study found that heavy meat-eaters were twice as likely to become demented over time than vegetarians of similar ages, genders and zip codes. And the age at which one is diagnosed with dementia is greatly delayed for vegetarians as well.[44] (P. Giem et al, 1993,) How is this possible?

A plant-heavy diet lowers your risk of high blood pressure, heart disease and diabetes, all of which are risk factors for dementia.[45] (Wei Xu et al, 2015.) In a review of the big three Adventist studies in America:

> . . .both lacto-ovo-vegetarians and vegans have reduced risk for hypertension, Type 2 diabetes, and obesity; however, vegans experienced greater risk reduction for those diseases. Similarly, both lacto-ovo-vegetarian males and vegan male have lower mortality from cardiovascular disease compared to non-vegetarians, but risk reduction is greater among vegans." [46] (Lap Tei Le et al, 2014.)

In other words, the more of your plate you cover in plants, the higher the levels of protection. Or as Walter Willet from the

Harvard School of Public health puts it: "Meat is like radiation: we don't know the safe level." Best to avoid it altogether.[47] *(www.hsph.Harvard.edunutritionsource/.)*

Need a little more proof? Here is a fantastic study coming out of Finland called "The FINGER Study." The Finnish Geriatric Intervention Study to Prevent Cognitive Impairment and Disability, which somehow spells FINGER as their acronym, is a two-year-long, double-blind randomized control trial looking at whether or not modifying the modifiable risk factors for cognitive decline would, in fact, reduce the risk of cognitive decline. Two groups were randomized either to receive help with their diet, exercise, cognitive training and vascular risk monitoring or just to receive general health advice. The recommended diet was heavy in whole grains, fruits, vegetables and plant-based oils, and participants were encouraged to greatly reduce or avoid milk and meat products. After two years, the intervention group scored better on their mental screening tests than the control group. Most notably, there were substantial improvements in the patients' executive functions and processing speed.[48] *(Tia Ngandu et al, 2015.)*

This study to me points out two things. Number one: a program that attacks multiple problems at once works. Number two: trusting status quo health advice does not work. To alter your health and cheat your genetic destiny, you have to color outside the lines. As the old saying goes: "Any cold, dead fish can float downstream. Only a live, healthy fish can fight against the current, swim up the waterfalls and avoid the bears." Said another way, if you eat, drink, and act like everyone else, do not be shocked when you end up just as sick as everyone else.

The other good thing about the FINGER study is that the intervention arm worked for all participants regardless of where they were on the socioeconomic ladder, how healthy or sick they were, or really what age or even gender they were.[49] *(Anna Rosenberg et al, 2018.)* This type of program works for everyone.

How To

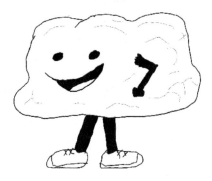

This book is not meant to exhaustively describe my years of research; neither will it be full of anecdotes. I envision this as a field guide, not an encyclopedia. The idea is to lay out a program that could be started today with no fancy or expensive extras.

Therefore, we will not spend a great deal of time arguing over competing theories. Those books are out there, and I welcome you to read them. You'll enjoy it even better after you've tuned your brain up with this program. But be careful! There is so much junk science and loud noise out there, especially on the Internet and social media sites. Some of it is, I hope, well intentioned. Some is being produced by folks who stand to profit from the status quo. For example, for years the cigarette industry pumped out numerous studies extolling the many positive medical benefits from smoking. While audacious, that's not completely untrue: smoking does help the symptoms of Parkinson's disease, as well as irritable bowel syndrome. But, of course, those meager benefits are greatly overshadowed by dying from lung cancer or COPD. Did the tobacco company executives want their customers to get cancer? Probably not. At least, I hope not. But the Tobacco Barons definitely wanted their customers to continue buying cigarettes so they could keep making money from those sales.

It is impossible to completely remove a person's bias, especially when that person is passionate about the subject being discussed. But I have done my best to showcase only what has been shown to work. And by "work," I mean not merely reducing the potential risk factors for dementia. I mean helping people truly avoid the disease. And if a patient already has dementia, let's slow the beast down, or even stop it in its tracks.

I'm not that interested in the studies showing that Such-N-Such Compound successfully treated Alzheimer's in mice. Partly I'm not interested because I do not treat mice and rats. If you are reading this book, you are not a rat, you are a human, and that is the group we need to treat. Rat studies are not that interesting to me because Alzheimer's in rats is quite easy to treat. Just throw some blueberries at them and their little brains get better. [50] *(Hai-Qiang Lee, et al, 2020.)* Throwing blueberries at human dementia patients doesn't work quite so well.[51] *(Erin L. Boespflug et al, 2018.)* Again, no silver bullets, no one magic capsule. It takes a multi-pronged attack to produce results.

I also want you to get started today with minimal stuff. I don't want you to have to wait for your specialized piece of equipment or your magic pills from the moons of Pluto to arrive before you get started. This program can be started when you are halfway through the book. Please read the whole book to get the whole program, but you get the idea.

Plus, I want this program to be for everyone. In the back of the book, there are a few supplements I will recommend. Some are inexpensive; some are not. But the supplements to the program are just that: supplemental. This whole program is based on what you can do to shift your brain from a destructive mode into a healing mode. It is not based on what you can take. You are probably taking too many pills as it is. Why add to the pile unnecessarily? If you follow this program, you will be shedding pharmaceutical pills anyway, as your brain and your body get healthier and healthier. You can do 90 percent of this program and get a huge amount of benefit with nothing more than a grocery cart full of healthy food, a pair of walking shoes, and a rope. No weird tests, no weird IVs, no special concoctions.

I will only recommend therapies and strategies that are mostly gain, very little pain. Example: Some data suggest coconut oil can be good for Alzheimer's, however there is a good deal of data suggesting it is bad for heart disease and diabetes. We are here to help the brain, but not at the expense of any of the other organ systems.

We will be discussing coconut oil, the possible benefits as well as the potential risks in the Supplements section later in the book. That way you are free to decide what would be the best choice for you and your situation.

Diet

We know that the standard American diet--high fat, high sugar, with little to no veggies or fruits--is associated with memory loss, a smaller hippocampus and a shrinking brain.[52] *(Felice N. Jacka et al, 2015.)* A chilling trial from 2017 showed that just four days of a breakfast high in saturated fat and added sugar has a negative impact on hippocampal-based learning.[53] *(Tuki Attuquayefio et al, 2017.)* In neurology, we use MRI studies to determine the size of the hippocampus, a way to find out if the patient has Alzheimer's. The smaller the hippocampus, the better chance your patient has Alzheimer's disease. This type of study fuels rants at my patients when I hear their favorite breakfast is microwaveable frozen sausages wrapped in pancakes soaked in syrup.

The stuff you put at the end of your fork is one of the most important choices any of us can make. We are literally what we eat. Every day your body's cells are repaired, rebuilt or replaced. Where does all of the raw material for that repair work come from? The food we eat. So, we get the wonderful opportunity to choose what type of building material we want to use each day to build our bodies. Let us then choose wisely. The first and most important pillar this program is built upon is diet.

Too many people are probably going to skip this section and head straight for the supplements section. That would be a mistake. I have seen far too many patients come in with memory loss taking pages of "all natural" pills and concoctions. All to no avail. Remember, they are called "supplements" because they are supplemental to The Main Thing. And The Main Thing is the food we eat. Everything else revolves around this central pillar.

As of this writing, a search for "diet books" on Amazon yields more than 60,000 results. How in the world can anyone choose the best plan out of 60,000 options? To narrow down the field, let's focus on our three top contributors to dementia: Inflammation & Rust, Plumbing Clogs, & Sugar Problems. We want to choose foods that will effectively deal with all three.

Cool the inflammation and stop the rust

Oxidation is a fancy term for rusting. And unless you are an interior decorator trying to add rustic charm to your new kitchen remodel, it is always a bad thing. As we discussed previously, just as your apple turns brown and goes bad if left out on the counter, so will your brain if it is unprotected from oxidation. And no one wants a brown, mushy brain. This oxidative stress, this rusting of your insides, leads to inflammation. And inflammation leads to high blood pressure, vascular disease, and dementia. The foods we choose must fight against oxidation and inflammation. And diets that are rich in fruits and vegetables do just that. The polyphenols found in fruits and vegetables are powerful antioxidants.[54] *(Yu-Chen Cheng et al, 22017.)* And a diet rich in antioxidants from fruits, vegetables, as well as whole grains, and even chocolate (!) has been found to lower the risk of stroke.[55] *(Susanne Rautiainen et al, 2012.)* (Go ahead and dip that apple slice into the chocolate hummus and live a little!!)

You will find a few supplements in the back of the book that can also help reduce inflammation in the body. Again, they are supplemental to the main program. A few herbs alone ain't going to cut it.

Clean the gunk out of the pipes and let the blood flow

As you learned earlier, atherosclerosis and dementia are quite firmly linked.[56] *(Alex E. Roher et al, 2011.)* Clogged-up pipes will not only kill off your heart muscle, but damage your brain tissue as well. So, what we eat has to help with inflammation and prevent cholesterol from gunking up your arteries. There are many foods to choose that have been shown to reduce the risk factors for heart attacks, and strokes. But why settle for a diet that *might* help reduce the risk of atherosclerosis? Why not go straight for a way of eating proven multiple times over multiple decades to reverse heart disease and open up clogged arteries?[57] *(Dean Ornish et al,1990.)*

Sure, there are plenty of ways to eat that will lead to a significant weight loss. But we are not looking to get you back into your old high school prom dress or tux. There is only one diet that has been proven to reverse heart disease by opening arteries all over the body. And keeping them open and happy for years.[58] *(Caldwell B. Esselstyn, Jr. et al, 2014.)* We want to save your brain, save your life, not merely have you look good at your high school reunion. A whole-food, plant-based diet has been shown again and again to halt the progression of heart disease. Remember, the idea is not just to keep your arteries from getting worse, but actually help them get better.[59] *(Dean Ornish et al, 1998.)*

The Nurses' Health Study showed an inverse relationship between fruit and vegetable intake and heart disease. Again, thank our friend polyphenols. Each additional serving of leafy green vegetables per day resulted in an 11 percent decreased risk for heart disease.[60] *(Hsin-Chia Hung et al, 2004.)* Leafy greens help to repair endothelial function in arteries.[61] *(Phillip Tuso et al, 2015.)* What the heck is that? Think of a Slip-and-Slide. As a kid, you wanted a nice smooth ride down the slide to the bottom, right? Rocks, sticks, gravel were a surefire way to reduce the safety and certainly the enjoyment of your experience. And so it is within your arteries. Your red blood cells want a nice smooth ride. And the inner lining of your arteries, the endothelial cells, are needed to provide that smooth ride. But you need miles and miles of smooth, gravel-free endothelial cells. We have roughly 60,000 miles of arteries according to Google. Cheese-burgers and hotdogs injure your endothelial cells.[62] *(Alicia Wolk, 2017.)* Eating them is like tossing rocks on the Slip-and-Slide. Don't do it.

With a plant-heavy diet, your arteries, suddenly healthy and happy, will start to open up, bringing blood to starving cells all over your body, including your brain. Starved brain cells drink deep and start to get healthy again. And healthy brain cells are what we are after with this program.

Call Roto-Rooter…

Stop gunk from clogging up your arteries, and while you're at it get good relief from the crippling symptoms of advanced heart disease. Who doesn't want that? And what do you eat on a Whole Plant Food Diet? Plenty of tasty fruits, veggies, beans and healthy starches that keep you satisfied, happy, and full of energy, all the while reversing the number-one killer of men and women world-wide.[63] *(Caldwell B. Esselstyn, Jr, et al, 1999,)* When we are looking for the diet that will give our brains the very best chance of recovery, why mess around with anything other than a sure thing? And, by the way, now you will have found a great way to fit back into your old prom dress (or tux, as the case may be).[64] *(Michael Greger, 2020.)*

Why not just follow your cardiologist's advice and go with the American Heart Association's recommended diet? It's ok, and anything is better than eating a double bacon, egg, and cheese-burger. But the AHA diet doesn't reduce your body's levels of inflammation as well as a plant-based diet does. The plant-based diet also lowers LDL cholesterol more than the AHA diet does.[65] *(Binita Shah et al, 2018.)*

36

Why can't we go on a Paleo diet or even Keto to solve the problem? Because the type of fat we eat makes a difference in how our brains work. The Harvard Women's study found the higher intake of saturated fat (mostly from meat and dairy) to be significantly associated "with worse global cognitive and verbal memory trajectories" over just a five-year period. Intake of monounsaturated fats was linked to "better trajectories." In plain English, women in the study had as much as a 70 percent greater chance of cognitive deterioration with a high intake of the type of fat found in meat and dairy products. Women with lower amounts of saturated fat and higher amounts of the type of fats found in nuts, seeds and other plants had brains that functioned six years younger on average.[66] *(Olivia I. Okereke et al, 2012.)*

Reverse your diabetes, improve your brain

Diabetes runs in my family over the river and through the woods to the grandparents' house. Aunts and uncles on both my mom's side and my dad's side dealt with it. My dad and brother wrestle with it. "Having a touch of the sugars," as my older patients call it, is blamed on genetics. In my twenties, I started passing out if my blood sugar got too low. There is a great story from my college days. I was working backstage at a musical and not paying attention to what or if I had been eating that day. I started getting woozy-headed and had just enough time to warn one of the beautiful dancing girls, "I'm going to pass out on you now." I then proceeded to collapse my 220-pound frame on top of the poor girl.

Waking up on the floor with people staring down at you asking what is wrong is not a great feeling. I was shuffled off to the infirmary, diagnosed with low blood sugar and given a snack. Problem solved. I just had to keep eating. So, every three to four hours I would have a small snack. Unfortunately, my small snacks kept getting bigger. And bigger. At the same time, I kept getting bigger. And bigger.

In my thirties, I was diagnosed as prediabetic. I also had high cholesterol and high blood pressure. "OK," I said, "I'll just lose weight, and everything will be fine." So, I did. I had already lost more than 60 pounds on Weight Watchers after graduating college. I looked good, but still had high blood pressure and cholesterol problems. I got back on the bandwagon. Ate less, exercised more. Got down to my perfect BMI and achieved Weight Watchers' Lifetime Member status. Conventional wisdom says that should have fixed everything, right? It did not. Even after having lost 80 pounds, I was still plagued with what is affectionately called "The Metabolic Syndrome": a potent mix of high blood pressure, high cholesterol and above average blood sugars, which doubles your risk of heart disease and causes a 1.5-fold increase in all causes of mortality. [67] *(Salvatore Mottillo et al, 2010.)* As a day-to-day aggravation, I was still having blood sugar problems, still getting woozy and dizzy if I went more than four hours without food. Clearly, I thought, this is genetic, and I'm doomed.

The single change I made that impacted my health the most was to quit focusing on how much food was on my plate for weight loss, but instead changing what was on my plate for health. Quickly after I switched to a whole-food plant diet, my high blood pressure disappeared, my bad cholesterol sank like a stone, my good cholesterol rose to unseen heights and my blood sugars comfortably nestled in the low end of normal. I can now go for hours and hours without eating, having completed multiple 24-hour-water-only fasts with no problems. Doomed by genetics? No. I had been doomed by my food choices. Just because I was eating smaller amounts of crap than I had when I was obese doesn't mean I wasn't still eating crap.

I ♥ Carbs

How do you lose weight and potentially completely reverse your diabetes eating carbohydrate-loaded beans, bananas and potatoes? Everyone "knows" carbs are the enemy and they will make you fat, diabetic and dead.

Ask anyone who is diabetic, or has lived with a diabetic, what happens when you eat a banana? They will tell you their blood sugars skyrocket. Case closed.

Or is it?

Why does the banana make the blood sugar go up? You eat the banana, your wonderful digestive system breaks down the fruit into its basic components until you are left with glucose, the body's preferred fuel source.[68] *(John T. Brosnan, 1999.)* In diabetic patients, the glucose floats around in the bloodstream, building up because it has nowhere to go due to problems with insulin. In Type 1 diabetes, this is due to a lack of enough insulin. In Type 2 diabetes, the sugar build-up is due to a lack of insulin's function.

Type 1 diabetes can certainly benefit from eating a Whole Food Plant Diet, but most Americans are at risk of or are already suffering from Type 2, so we will concentrate on that for now.

Let's start with the most basic of biology questions: What does insulin do?

A quick refresher of your 8th grade biology: Every cell in your body runs on sugar. It's the preferred fuel source. Yes, we are fearfully and wonderfully made, thus we have back-up systems that can be used when needed. But if you ask your muscle cells what they want the most for Christmas, they are going to tell Santa sugar. How does the sugar get from the banana into the hungry muscle cell? Insulin is released when we eat. Every time we eat. It has to be, since insulin is the only way that glucose can get into all of your body's cells.

It is an elegant lock-and-key mechanism. On the outside of all the cells in your body there is a special lock, officially called an "insulin receptor." All the cells in your body have one. (Ok, maybe not your fingernails, but you get the idea.) You eat the banana, your body does a fancy hokey-pokey style dance called the "Krebs Cycle," and you get glucose. Now, the glucose needs somewhere to go. Insulin is released by the pancreas, and heads toward your muscle cell. The key--insulin--slides into the insulin receptor in the cell wall, the lock, and your cell wall opens up like unto Pac Man and starts to gobble up the glucose pellets as they go by. Mealtime over, insulin is removed from the lock, and the cell wall closes back up to prevent any bad guys from getting in. Muscles are happy, glucose levels back to normal, and you are ready to go climb that tree.

So why did our diabetic from before have such trouble with the banana? It's not the insulin's fault. Remember, insulin is released every time we eat, no matter what we eat. It is possible to proportionally release just as much insulin from eating steak as you can from eating pasta.[69] *(Susanne H. Holt et al, 1997.)* Type 2 diabetes is caused by the failure of insulin to function. The insulin gets less and less effective, causing the body to release more insulin, which continues to not work. Insulin levels rise, the muscle cells can't get the glucose they are craving and the blood sugar starts to sky rocket. So why does the insulin stop working? We need to go a few steps deeper, to get at the root cause of high insulin levels: intramyocellular lipid content. Not only is that a guaranteed winning word at Scrabble, it is a huge contributor to diabetes. An abundance of evidence suggests triglycerides and fat have a causal relationship with insulin resistance and diabetes.[70] *(J. Denis McGarry, 2002.)*

Fat builds up inside your muscle cells, causing inflammation, and free radical damage, preventing insulin from doing its job. Within five days of your starting a high-fat diet, researchers have found your ability to process glucose is reduced by 50 percent![71] *(Michael Roden et al, 1996.)* Within hours of ingesting fat, your body's ability to handle glucose is compromised.[72] *(Michael Roden et al, 1999.)* The inflammation from a high-fat diet damages the body's cell, which allows fat to accumulate inside the cell, where it ought not be.[73] *(Dawn K. Coletta et al, 2011.)* Like a well-marbled steak, the fat builds up. The key would still work, it's just that the lock gets clogged up with fat. As the lock gets clogged up, your body releases more and more insulin to try and get the same response. As the insulin begins to lose its function, the sugar starts to back up, and you start to become more and more diabetic.

Not all fats end up marbling muscle cells. Saturated fat, found mostly in meat, dairy and eggs, causes a toxic soup called "lipotoxicity," leading first to fat's becoming embedded in the cell wall and thence leading to intramyocellular lipids, after that to insulin resistance, and finally to diabetes. Monounsaturated fat, found mostly in nuts, olives and avocados, has been found to be protective against the damage from saturated fat.[74] *(Christopher J. Nolan et al, 2009.)* Muscle biopsies show that as the saturated fat builds up in muscle cells, insulin resistance rises.[75] *(Gianluca Perseghin et al, 1999.)* On the other hand, monounsaturated fats/plant fats, are safely tucked away in fat cells where they belong, or just get detoxified and pass.[76] *(Christopher J. Nolan et al, 2009.)*

This was my path to diabetes. My well-marbled muscles, full of fat, were leading to a nice liver full of fat, which would push me all the way over into pure diabetes. Removing the saturated fat from my diet, coupled with exercise, burned the gunk out of my cellular locks, allowing my insulin to function normally again and dropping my blood sugar into normal levels. Therefore, let us correct the underlying problem of insulin resistance--intramyocellular lipids. Then we can supplement with ketone salts if needed.[77] *(Suzanne M. de la Monte, 2014.)*

Why not meat?

The better question is, "why meat?"

> *"Someone asked me how could you get as strong as*
> *an ox without eating meat? My answer was, 'have*
> *you ever seen an ox eating meat? '"* –**Patrik**
> **Baboumian**, *vegan strongman and bodybuilder*

It is a tightly held and long-fought-over myth that there is something magical about the protein or nutrients in animal muscle tissue. This is false. Animal-based proteins are not superior to the proteins found in plants. A strong argument can be made that the proteins found in meat originally came from plants, since that's what the cow/sheep/chicken was eating before you barbequed its shoulder muscle and plopped it on your plate.

Let's look at the biggest, strongest animals, like rhinos, elephants and gorillas. No one is asking the Silverback gorilla where he is getting his protein. Elephants aren't worried about trying to combine the correct kind of amino acids; they just eat their plants and keep rolling. That's what I do, and that's what I encourage you to do. A plant-based diet easily gives you all the amino acids you need to keep your body strong while improving your mind. A plant-based diet gives you all the vitamins and minerals you need, except for B12.

What About B12?

B12 is essential to brain and nerve health. Most people get it from eating meat, but its original source is soil bacteria. The cow or pig grabs a mouthful of grass and some dirt, and Voila! gets some free B12. The B12 gets stored and shows back up in your hamburger later. We do not recommend eating more dirt to raise your B12 levels for three reasons:

1. It's gross.
2. It will not work. There is less and less B12 in the soil due to our use of pesticides and the general poor condition of our soil. Therefore, your cows and pigs aren't getting as much as they used to, so even in your pork chops there's less B12 than there used to be.
3. There's a better way. Just pop a tiny pill.

We will be recommending B12 supplementation later in the supplements section. As we all get older, we absorb less and less B12 from our food. Most of my patients over the age of 70 require B12 supplementation of some kind, whether they are vegetarians or carnivores.

"But that guy at the gym told me that cholesterol is good for you, and I need to take these amino acids pills."

Cholesterol is vital to the body. Your brain and cell membranes are made of cholesterol. It is so vital, so important to the human body your liver makes all you will ever need. We don't need to eat more.

And as to taking amino acid pills or eating meat to stave off nutrient deficiency: gym rats also boast about a few nutrients touted as uniquely found in animals, which is also false. These nutrients, like taurine or creatine, are made in your liver whenever your body needs them. So long as you eat enough calories on a plant-based diet, you will get more than enough protein, and the proper mix of amino acids as well. Most of the research that tells you to consume a specific substance to optimize health is done by folks trying to sell you that substance.

"But that guy at the gym told me cholesterol doesn't cause heart attacks."

Biff might be right. He might also be horribly wrong. There is significant, knife-wielding controversy on that fact. Scientists, medical doctors and journalists are constantly fighting each other over it.

Why take the chance? Again, there is not anything other than B12 that you could get from animals that you can't get from plants. And with plants, you get bonus items, like fiber, phytonutrients, vitamins and minerals. We are trying to optimize your brain's chances of healing itself. Why do anything that might raise your risk of having a stroke and further injure the brain we are fighting to protect?

Again, the whole plant diet has been proven time and time again to promote incredible health and reverse some of our most debilitating diseases, even heart disease. And since there is nothing superior to plants in the animal kingdom, the question remains: Why meat? Sure, it has protein, but that protein comes mixed with a giant wad of unhealthy fats, and carcinogens. Just eat what elephants eat and get healthy.

What About Fish?

Most folks believe they need to eat fish for heart and brain health. However, mercury, lead and other brain toxins are almost impossible to avoid in any fish you buy from the store or catch in the river.[78] *(Adina E Bosch et al, 2016.)* This goes back to our principle of *Do No Harm*. The brain-healthy goodness from fish often comes wrapped in a brain toxin burrito.[79] *(Jin-Ling Lu et al, 2015.)*

The authors discussing the benefits of fish are all using short-term studies. But we know for a fact that long-term lead and mercury consumption is terrible for long-term brain health. Why do you think it is recommended that pregnant ladies forego seafood? It's bad for developing baby brains. But the toxins in seafood never stop being dangerous. We should all be avoiding them on a regular basis, especially if you are concerned with dementia. We are trying to flush more and more toxins out of the body, so why risk adding more?

All the healthy components of fish, DHEA, ALA, etc., can be found in the plant kingdom, from walnuts, broccoli and algae. Where do you think the fish get their DHEA? We will discuss fish oil supplements in more detail in the supplement section later on in the book. Spoiler alert: you might be wasting your money.[80] *(Akshay Goel et al, 2018.)*

Not All or Nothing

Not everyone can go cold turkey overnight on a plant-based diet and make it stick. My wife and I couldn't. We tried a couple of times. What worked was setting small changes, small goals and achieving them. Then making some more small changes, new slightly bigger goals and achieving those goals. This will build in your new way of eating bit by bit, brick by brick until it is a cozy, warm house of health.

Multiple studies have shown that even baby steps toward a plant-based diet pay good dividends.[81] *(Gina Segovia-Siapco et al,*

2019.) Replacing the puny scrap of grilled chicken on your salad with a giant mound of chickpeas is a wonderful change that will start to move your body into a healing mode. And as the body goes, the mind follows.

Blue Zones

Yes, I'm talking about the Blue Zones again. The book you might want to read after this one is called *The Blue Zones*, by Dan Buetner. He can thank me later for referring to it again. This information was originally from a National Geographic study on the places in the world with the highest levels of centenarians (people who live to 100 years or more). At the time of the study, there were five areas, dubbed Blue Zones, in the world:

- The Italian island of Sardinia
- Okinawa, Japan
- Loma Linda, California
- Costa Rica's isolated Nicoya Peninsula
- Ikaria, an isolated Greek island

People in these areas ate a diet high in complex carbohydrates, lower in protein and low in fat. Roughly 95 percent of their diet came from plants of all kinds. In some of the zones people loved beans a little more than others, some loved sweet potatoes, but throughout they were mostly plant-based. Not 100 percent. Some ate goat cheese a few times a week, or literally killed the fatted calf or goat for celebrations a few times a year. Small pockets of meat consumption here and there surrounded by days and weeks of plant-heavy plates--the exact opposite of how most Americans and people in other western countries eat. And the extended healthy life spans in the blue zones show the difference.

Daily activity was also one of the findings the folks in each zone shared. We will discuss this further in the exercise section.

I mention the blue zones to point out that the goal is not 1000 percent perfection. That is not only mathematically impossible, it's ridiculous to expect anyone, including me, to pull it off.

Flip the Plate

The goal is to choose foods that are nourishing for your body, your gut, and your brain. All positives, no negatives. And we want to succeed in creating an ultimate goal such as: "This is how we are going to eat five years from now."

Dr. Garth Davis in his book, *Proteinaholic*, talks with his patients about "flipping the plate." I find this strategy works well with my patients also. I live and work in Alabama, and my patients know what a "Meat & Three" place is--usually a cafeteria-style restaurant where your meal is a slab of some type of meat--ham, turkey, hamburger steak, fried chicken--followed by three different, much smaller sides: mac-n-cheese, mashed potatoes, fried okra, etc. I tell them to flip the plate, get three large servings of sides, mostly vegetables, and a small serving of meat. Usually the patient relaxes, smiles and says, "OK, I can do *that*." It's a great place to start.

Tortoise and Hare

Remember, the goal is a happy, healthy brain and body. While we want to reach that goal as fast as we can, we need to retool our idea of what it will look like in real life. This will not be like getting to the end of a diet, looking good during our beach vacation and then going back to business as usual. No. Business as usual is how we got to this point in the first place. The goal here is to have as healthy a brain as we can by implementing the strategies in this book. And then continuing them for at least another 20 years or until something better comes along. And since there is nothing better on the horizon, we had better buckle down for the long haul.

Organic vs Regular

A common question is whether organic produce is worth the extra money. A quick Google search will give you 656,000,000 different opinions, mostly from people wanting to sell you stuff. The scientific literature is a bit more nuanced than the hippie at the farmers' market braiding his hair while telling you conventionally grown tomatoes will kill you.

There is not that much evidence that the organically grown produce is significantly more nutritious than the conventionally grown produce.[82] *(Faidon Magkos et al, 2003.)*

But while they might not have more Vitamin C, organic fruits and vegetables do have less pesticide residue than conventionally grown produce. The levels of exposure for both conventional and organic are still low per tomato, but what we would worry about is the cumulative buildup over time.[83] *(Faidon Magkos et al, 2006.)*

Same problem with heavy toxic metals in our soil and in fertilizers. The toxic heavy metal cadmium can be found in both conventional and organic food, but the levels are much lower in the organic produce.[84] *(Anna Lindén et al, 2001.)* So, a diet that favors more organic produce over time will have less pesticide residue and heavy metals than the conventional produce.

Does that equate to less cancer? Maybe, maybe not. A study of more than 600,000 UK women followed for more than nine years found no significant difference between the rates of cancer diagnosis in those associated with eating organic produce and those who did not. There was a slight bump in non-Hodgkin's lymphoma cases, otherwise no real difference.[85] *(K. E. Bradbury et al, 2014.)*

A paper published in 2011 links pesticide exposure in foods to testicular cancer, though the main source of the pesticides was in high-fat dairy products, not produce.[86] *(Fabrizio Giannandrea et al, 2011.)* And then there is an unintentionally amusing study that found fruit flies fed a diet of organic bananas, potatoes, raisins and soybeans did better than flies given conventional produce. The organically fed fruit flies not only lived longer, but exhibited better stress resistance and increased fertility. This is believed to be due to the lower amount of pesticides in the food, which of course only makes sense. Fruit flies fed a diet lower in pesticides designed to kill them do better than those that aren't.[87] *(Ria Chhabra et al, 2013.)*

For those of us who are not fruit flies, is organic produce worth the extra money? I'll give you a very firm "maybe." The danger from putting organic foods on a high pedestal of righteousness derives from the risk that people think organic is the only option, but they can't afford it, and give up and go back to eating 99-cent cheeseburgers.

So, my recommendation is if you can afford the organic produce, great. If not, still fill your grocery cart with all the brain-saving plant-powered nutrition you can. If everyone in America would add just one serving of fruits and vegetables a day, it is estimated approximately 20,000 cancer cases per year could be prevented. Twenty thousand! And that's using conventional produce. The downside? There could be 10 cancer cases a year possibly caused by the pesticide consumption.[88] *(Richard Reiss et al, 2012.)* I think preventing 19,990 cases of cancer is worth the risk.

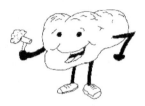 # Recipes

What in the world is that?

Before we begin, there are a few items in these recipes that my family and I tend to take for granted, but I thought it might be useful to explain what they are, and why we use them in our recipes.

- **Nutritional Yeast**: Nooch! Magic Cheeto Dust! Hippie Dust! Beloved of vegans everywhere, nutritional yeast is a deactivated yeast used as a cheese substitute in numerous plant-based recipes due to its cheesy, umami flavor. The most common form looks like golden fish food, though I have seen some that is more granular. It is a great source of all nine essential amino acids & protein, along with B vitamins and other minerals. It even has four grams of fiber in two tablespoons. It is often used in recipes, but we also sprinkle it on darn near everything.

- **Miso Paste:** a salty, savory paste used in Japanese cuisine for centuries. The base is fermented soybeans with additional ingredients almost individualized per producer. High in protein, and chock full of vitamins and minerals, it comes in a variety of shades of color and flavor.

- **Tahini:** A paste made from ground sesame seeds, it has been used in Middle Eastern and North African cuisines for centuries. Not quite as savory as miso, tahini is one of the main ingredients in hummus. Since it is mostly ground seeds, half of its calories come from fat, the other half split almost evenly between carbohydrates and protein.

- **Tamari:** Basically a gluten/wheat-free version of soy sauce. I find it has a deeper, richer flavor, which is why I prefer it. If you can't find it, or don't want to look because you already have a bottle of Kikkoman, feel free to use soy sauce.

- **Bragg's Liquid Aminos:** Another gluten-free alternative to soy sauce. A little thinner, slightly sweeter, but with less preservatives than most commercial soy sauces. It's also kosher. (הנאה!) Do not be fooled, liquid aminos and tamari are still full of sodium, just like soy sauce. So don't drown your food in it thinking just because it is slightly more exotic it's magically healthier.

- **Almond milk versus soy milk versus oat milk:** Each nondairy milk has a slightly different flavor, which can be helpful or almost necessary depending upon what recipe you are using. No surprise, almond has a slightly nutty taste. Oat milk for my money is the creamiest. For recipes, soy is pretty neutral, and it goes with everything. The most important thing to know when using plant-based milks is that most of them are sweetened. This makes them taste better in your cereal or coffee. However, I have learned the hard way that using a sweet milk can ruin a savory recipe. What we do at my house: use the regular slightly sweeter milks and buy a carton that explicitly says unsweetened for cooking.

Cashew Cheese Sauce

This sauce is awesome for pasta, potatoes, pizza base, rice and veggie bowls, basically anything to which you want to add cheese. It's great for dipping crusty bread, too. My son, Noah, is my picky eater, and he loves this sauce. He especially likes to mix it with marinara sauce to take spaghetti over the top!

*adapted from *This Cheese is Nuts* by Julie Piatt

- 1 cup raw cashews, soaked overnight in water OR soaked 20 min in boiling hot water
- 1/4 chickpea miso (found at Whole Foods)
- 1 Tbsp nutritional yeast
- 1 Tbsp lemon juice
- 1/2 tsp garlic powder
- 1/2 tsp salt
- 1 cup boiling water (not for soaking)

In a high-speed blender, blend all ingredients on medium for 1-2 minutes. If you do not soak the cashews, you will be dealing with a grittier texture so make sure you soak. If you do not have a Vitamix, soak overnight, covered in the fridge.

This recipe will cover a pound of pasta very nicely. Feel free to add a can of peas if your kid will eat it with that addition. Or try lightly steamed broccoli.

Almond Cheddar Spread/Dip/Cheese Ball

I love the simplicity of this recipe. It has been adapted from *This Cheese is Nuts* by Julie Piatt. I admire her book, and this is one of several of her recipes we use religiously. It's a big hit at every party as a dip, it works great as a spread on sandwiches and wraps, and it can be formed into a cheeseball with crushed nuts covering the outside. I have made this recipe a little simpler, but notes below will tell you the original plan.

Spread

- 2 cups raw almonds
- 1 jar (7-oz) jar of pimentos, undrained
- 1/4 cup nutritional yeast
- 1 tsp salt
- 1 tsp garlic powder

Add everything to a Vitamix blender (pimentos first) and blend until smooth. Add water as needed to achieve desired consistency.

Cheeseball

Try not to add any water so the ball is as firm as possible. Empty the cheese onto a piece of waxed paper and form the ball. Crush a cup of toasted almonds or use toasted slivered almonds and press into the ball. Place on serving tray and add crackers or cut carrots and celery.

Note: If you do not have a Vitamix or other high-speed blender, soak the almonds overnight in water or soak in boiling hot water for 10 minutes. The original recipe uses 1 3/4 tsp smoked sea salt, so that's a cool spin you might try, too.

Caesar Dressing

My wife loves Caesar dressing. I like it, too. Not just because it's delicious, but because Caesar salads are always drowning in dressing. I hadn't been able to enjoy it in a while, because I don't want the high-fat, dairy options that are out there. A lot of the vegan options use vegan mayonnaise, which I have and use sparingly on sandwiches. It's so high in fat that I try to limit my use. So, when my wife found this recipe in the *Straight Up Food* cookbook, we got super excited! This is my wife's version of their recipe. Still unprocessed and you can feel good about loading the salad!

*adapted from *Straight Up Food Cookbook*
Makes 1 cup

- 1/2 cup water
- 1/2 cup raw, unsalted cashews
- 2 Tbsp lemon juice
- 2 Tbsp mustard (Dijon or stone ground)
- 1 date
- 1 prune (or in place of date and prune you can use 1 Tbsp raisins)
- 2 cloves garlic
- 1 tsp Italian herb seasoning
- 1 tsp garlic powder

Place all the dressing ingredients in a blender and set aside for 15 minutes (so cashews can soften, but you can bypass this step if you have a high-speed blender like Vitamix). Blend until smooth.

For a nut-free option, replace cashews with ¾ cup cooked or canned white beans.

Addicting Queso

You have been warned. This queso is off the charts. I'm not responsible for what I do with a pot of this and a bag of whole-grain Tostitos.

In a blender add:
- 2 cups water
- 1/3 cup nutritional yeast
- 1/4 cup Tahini
- 1/4 cup arrowroot powder or 7 tsp cornstarch
  (Both are gluten-free.)
- 2 Tbsp lemon juice
- 1 Tbsp onion powder
- 1 tsp salt
- 1 tsp cumin
- 1 tsp taco seasoning
- 2 dashes liquid smoke

Blend for a minute or two. Pour into a pot and add 1/2 can RoTel diced tomatoes and green chiles drained. (Your choice of original or mild.) Whisk rapidly over high heat until mixture thickens.
Eat entire pot in one sitting.

Sweet Potato Cheese Dip

Another cheese dip recipe? Yes. We are unapologetic about it. This can be made with sweet potatoes or with white potatoes if you don't want a hint of sweet.

- 1 large sweet potato, baked and peel removed
- 1.5 cups plant milk
- 1 cup nutritional yeast
- 1 tsp chili powder
- 1 tsp garlic powder
- 1 tsp onion powder
- 1 tsp smoked paprika
- 1 Tbsp Mike's seasoning, Lawry's salt, or Benson's Table Tasty for a sodium-free option
- 1 tsp sweet curry

Blend in a high-speed blender and warm in a microwave or on the stove.

Enjoy Raw Veggies Sauce

My wife and I ate a totally raw food diet for three weeks as an experiment. This sauce was one of the things that got me through it. Thank you to Chef AJ for the inspiration.

- 1 cup almond butter
- 1 cup coconut water
- ¼ cup lime juice
- 2 ½ tbsp tamari/soy sauce or Bragg's Liquid Aminos
- 4 pitted dates, soaked in water
- 3 cloves of garlic
- 1 inch fresh, peeled ginger
- ½ tsp red pepper flakes

Blend all ingredients in a high-speed blender until smooth and creamy. Smear on salads, wraps or anoint vegetables. I have not found anything that wasn't made better with this sauce.

White Bean Chili

Very satisfying, very filling chili. One of the true joys of plant-based eating is enjoying large portions. So go ahead, use the big bowl. You are welcome.

- 1 small yellow onion, diced
- Vegetable broth for sauté
- 3 cloves garlic, minced
- 1 1/2 tsp cumin
- 2 Tbsp tapioca flour
- 1 lb Yukon gold potatoes, chopped
- 4 cups vegetable broth
- 2 cans white beans, drained
- 1 cup corn kernels, canned or frozen
- 1 (16 oz) jar of salsa verde
- 1 (4 oz) can green chiles
- 1/2 tsp dried oregano
- salt and pepper to taste
- cilantro as an optional topping

In a large pot, sauté yellow onion until translucent. Add vegetable broth as the onion cooks to keep from sticking. Add garlic and cumin and sauté for 30 seconds, continuing to add broth as needed. Add tapioca flour, potatoes and 4 cups vegetable broth while stirring. Add white beans, corn, salsa verde, green chiles, and oregano. Let soup come to a boil and turn down to let simmer for 30 minutes so that potatoes cook. Stir frequently. Once potatoes are cooked, salt and pepper to taste.

Black-Eyed Pea and Greens Soup

*adapted from Carolyn Strickland a.k.a TofuChic

- 2 15-oz cans black-eyed peas, drained and rinsed
- ½ Tbsp extra virgin olive oil
- 1 large yellow onion, chopped
- 2 cloves garlic, finely chopped
- ½ package (two links) Field Roast Smoked Apple Sage "Sausage," sliced or diced
- 2 stalks celery, chopped
- 6 cups vegetable broth
- 1 large bunch kale, stems removed (also great with collards)
- 4 carrots, chopped
- ½ tsp liquid smoke
- ½ tsp smoked paprika

Heat oil in a skillet (or use some vegetable broth for an oil-free version). Cook sausage until lightly browned (2-3 min). Set aside in a bowl. In a stock pot over medium-high heat, sauté onion, garlic and celery until onion is translucent, typically 5-8 minutes, adding water a few tablespoons at a time to keep veggies from sticking to the pan. Add drained and rinsed black-eyed peas and broth and bring to a boil. Add carrots, liquid smoke, and paprika. (Add collards here, if using.) Simmer until tender, at least 20-30 minutes more. Add sausage and kale and simmer for 10 minutes.

Makes roughly 6 servings

Spicy Kale Salad Wrap

This can be used as a wrap or a topping to a salad or a large salad all by itself. It's chockful of flavor and pairs great with my wife's spicy radish microgreens!

Prep time: 25 minutes
Makes: 6 wraps

- 1 head of kale (finely chopped) or roughly half to 3/4 bag of organic kale
- 1/3 red onion (finely chopped) or about 1/2 cup
- 1 large avocado
- 1/2 c sun-dried tomatoes (from bag or jar), divided
- 1 Tbsp olive oil, or water for oil-free option
- 3 Tbsp nutritional yeast + an additional 4 Tbsp Nooch for the end
- 2 cloves garlic
- 2 Tbsp lemon juice
- 2 Tbsp tamari or Bragg's liquid aminos
- 1/2 bag of radish microgreens from Incredible Health Farms or local source
- 6 organic whole grain wraps

Blend olive oil or water, tamari, lemon juice, garlic cloves, 1/4 c chopped sundried tomatoes and three tablespoons nutritional yeast. Add more water if you need more liquid to blend. Remove kale from stems and chop finely. Chop radish and add to kale. Add red onion, avocado, 1/4 cup sundried tomatoes, blended mixture and four additional tablespoons of nutritional yeast. Massage everything together. (I recommend doing this part using disposable gloves.) Put roughly 1-2 cups in a wrap and enjoy!

BBQ Quinoa Bowl

This is one of Pop-Pop's favorite dishes, and an easy Go-To recipe in our house. I'm not sure how long it stays fresh in the fridge, since no matter how much I make it's gone by the next day. This is an adapted recipe from *Happy Herbivore*.

Make BBQ sauce and set aside to cool or use one cup commercial BBQ sauce free of high fructose corn syrup.

The BBQ Sauce part (makes 1 cup):
- 1/2 cup ketchup
- 1 Tbsp lemon juice
- 3 Tbsp apple cider vinegar
- 1 Tbsp vegan Worcestershire
- 1 Tbsp brown sugar
- 1 Tbsp Dijon mustard
- 1 tsp pepper
- 1 tsp smoked paprika or Smokehouse maple seasoning
- 1 tsp chili powder
- 1 tsp garlic powder
- 1 tsp onion powder
- 1/3 c water

In small saucepan combine all ingredients and whisk together while you bring the sauce to a boil. Reduce heat and simmer for 15 to 20 minutes.

The Quinoa and everything else part:
- 3 cups cooked quinoa
- 1 cup BBQ sauce
- 1 15-oz can black beans, rinsed and drained
- 10 oz cherry tomatoes
- 1 cup corn and/or chopped peppers (red, yellow and orange)
- 1/2 cup red onion
- Guacamole for an optional topping

Toss quinoa with BBQ sauce. Add beans, tomatoes, corn and/or peppers and onions. Mix together. Serve cold or warm topped with guacamole, which is recommended but not required.

Instant Pot Beans and Rice with Queso

Makes 6 to 8 servings

- 2 cups brown rice, any non-GMO brand
- 2 1/2 cups water or vegetable broth
- 2 cans beans, rinsed and drained (I prefer black, but use whatever makes you happy.)
- 2 cans Ro Tel, undrained
- 2 Tbsp garlic-and-herb seasoning
- 3 cups spinach, chopped, or ripped up with your hands right before tossing it in, like I do

Add all except spinach to an instant pot and set on manual for 25 minutes. When done, stir in spinach. It will wilt quickly. Serve in 2-cup servings topped with Addicting Queso.

Luck of the Irish Potatoes

Do not dishonor this dish by calling it merely "mashed potatoes." These are Irish potatoes and are far superior. Leeks can sometimes be hard to find, but they are worth the extra effort. This is supposed to be a side dish, but I have happily eaten it as my main meal. More than once. And I look forward to doing it again. So will you.

This recipe adapted from the *Plant Pure Nation* cookbook

- 6 medium potatoes, quartered
- ½ green cabbage, sliced into strips, the thinner, the better
- 1 onion, diced
- 2 leeks, chopped small
- 1 cup vegetable broth for sautéing the veggies
- ½ cup unsweetened non-dairy milk
- 4 Tbsp nutritional yeast flakes
- 3 Tbsp minced garlic
- 2 Tbsp chives or green onions
- 1 tsp salt
- 1 tsp black pepper

Throw the potatoes into a large pot, cover with water and boil until tender, not mushy. While the potatoes are cooking, sauté the cabbage, leeks, and onion using the veggie broth. (Remember, sautéing in broth reduces calories and oil, tastes the same and works just the same.) Cook until tender, drain.

In a bowl, mash the potatoes, adding the milk, garlic, nutritional yeast and chives. Fold in the cabbage and leeks and season with salt and pepper. Enjoy!

Can't find leeks? Use shallots or scallions. Can't find those? Just double the green onions instead.

Nothing Fishy Here Tacos

I used to love fish tacos, and now I can enjoy the same taste without all the mercury!

- One 15-oz can of chickpeas, rinsed and drained
- 1 tsp chili powder
- 3 cups shredded cabbage
- 1 cup shredded carrot
- ½ cup sliced red onion
- ½ cup chopped green onion
- ½ cup diced poblano peppers
- ¼ cup chopped fresh cilantro
- ½ cup vegan mayonnaise
- 2 Tbsp lime juice
- 1 tsp sea salt
- 1 avocado pitted and sliced
- Sriracha to taste
- 6 corn or flour tortillas

In a large bowl, mash the chickpeas with a fork while adding the chili powder. Then mix in the cabbage, carrots, red onion, poblano peppers, green onion, cilantro, lime juice and salt. Mix thoroughly. Divide among the tortillas. Crown each one with avocado slices and splash with Sriracha as desired.

Ridiculously Easy Black Bean Burgers

I often tell people how your taste for food changes, and you start to crave new comfort foods once you switch over to a plant-heavy diet. I love black bean burgers, and greatly prefer them to even Impossible or Beyond Beef burgers. This is a great quick recipe that we use when we have company over. We haven't had anyone yet turn her or his nose up at them. I know they last at least one day in the fridge, but they never stick around longer than that at our house.

This recipe doubles and even triples very well. *adapted with gratitude from *Happy Herbivore*

> Makes 4 burgers
> - 1 15-oz can organic black beans, drained and rinsed
> - 2 Tbsp organic ketchup
> - 1 Tbsp Dijon mustard
> - 1 tsp garlic powder
> - 1 tsp onion powder
> - 1 tsp Umami powder (Get yours at Trader Joe's or on Amazon.)
> - 3 drops of liquid smoke
> - ½ cup old fashioned oats

Preheat oven to 400 degrees and line a cookie sheet with parchment paper.

In a mixing bowl mash black beans with potato masher or fork until most of the beans are mashed up. Stir in condiments and spices; then fold in oats. Form the mixture into four patties and bake for 10 minutes. Carefully flip the burgers and bake another 5 minutes.

Kid Friendly Mac N Cheeze

*adapted from *Brand New Vegan*
Serves 4

This sauce is, for picky eaters like my son, a happy surprise. When it's left over, though, it does tend to be a little dry, so you might want to add a little vegan butter or unsweetened nondairy milk to thin it out again.

- 12-ounce box of macaroni noodles
   (whole wheat, or brown rice versions, your choice)
- 3 medium Yukon potatoes
- 7 to 8 oz carrots, chopped (about 1/2 of a 16-oz bag of baby carrots)
- 1/2 cup of water from the boiled potatoes
- 1/4 cup plus 2 Tbsp nutritional yeast
- 2 Tbsp lemon juice
- 1 tsp apple cider vinegar
- 1 tsp salt
- 1 tsp onion powder
- 1 tsp garlic powder
- 1 tsp brown mustard (or Dijon)
- 1/2 tsp turmeric

Wash and scrub potatoes and carrots; peel if you wish. Chop in uniform pieces and steam or boil in water for 10 minutes. Let rest for 5 minutes. Transfer veggies with a slotted spoon into the blender. Add ½ cup of the potato water. Pulse in blender. Add remaining ingredients and blend until smooth and creamy. Taste and add more salt if desired.

Boil noodles according to the package directions. Pour sauce over drained noodles and enjoy!

Make You Buff Beans and Greens

This recipe is one of my favorites in the whole book. It's adapted from Kim Campbell's wonderful version of Buffalo Beans and Greens. Her recipes are fantastic. I am deeply indebted. These beans are amazing. amazing. Looks weird, I know, but give it a chance.

- One 14-oz package of firm tofu, drained and cubed
- 1 cup buffalo wing sauce (Oil-free tastes brighter.)
- 1/2 tsp liquid smoke
- Two 15-oz cans of pinto or white beans, drained and rinsed
- 2 bunches of kale, sliced into strips with stems removed
- 4 cups of brown rice, cooked
- 1 ½ cup vegan bleu-cheese dressing (My wife prefers vegan ranch dressing.)

In a shallow dish, marinate the tofu in the buffalo sauce and liquid smoke for one hour. Preheat the oven to 375 degrees. Line a baking sheet with parchment paper. Remove the tofu from marinade and spread on the baking sheet. Bake for 15 minutes or until the edges are brown and dry. Turn over halfway through for best results.

Steam sliced kale in a small amount of water till wilted. Drain, then add the beans and mix together.

Add the rice to the plate, then add the kale/bean mixture and top with the tofu. Drizzle with the bleu-cheese dressing. Or ranch, if preferred. Add any extra buffalo sauce for taste or decoration as desired.

Butternut Squash Quinoa Casserole

This is a recipe we did in one of our meal-prep classes, Incredible Health Made Easy, which we hope to start back one day when the quarantine is over. The meals that were sent home with the customers received rave reviews, even by the husbands who had previously refused to eat plant-based dishes.

*modified from *trialandeater.com*

Servings 6 to 8 (6 if it's a meal, 8 if it's a side)

- 6 cups cubed butternut squash
- 1 cup uncooked quinoa + 2 cups water (makes 3 cups cooked quinoa)
- 1 can sweet corn, drained
- 1 can black beans, drained and rinsed
- 1 can diced tomatoes, drained (Fire-roasted work great.)
- 1 Tbsp cumin
- 1 lime, juiced (or 2 Tbsp bottled lime juice)
- 1 to 2 cups non-dairy cheddar cheese
- 1 avocado, diced
- salsa

Preheat oven to 400 degrees.

Steam 6 cups butternut squash. Meanwhile, bring 2 cups of water to a boil and add 1 cup quinoa. Simmer for 15 minutes or until water is absorbed.

In a 9x13 casserole dish add the cooked squash, corn, black beans, tomatoes, cumin, lime juice, salt and pepper and toss together. Top with quinoa and mix again.

Top with cheese and bake for 15 minutes or until cheese is melted. Top with avocado and spoonsful of salsa.

African Queen Stew

This recipe doubles really well, which is good, because you are going to want a second helping. You could eat this as a stand-alone stew and be happy, but it's part of my heritage to pour yummy stuff over rice to double the enjoyment. That's how I eat it; that's how I recommend eating it.

- 2 onions sliced into ¼ inch rings
- 2 celery stalks, diced
- 2 carrots, diced
- 2 sweet potatoes, cubed
- 3 tsp minced garlic
- 1 cup veggie stock
- One 28-oz can diced tomatoes
- 2 Tbsp curry powder
- 2 tsp sea salt
- 1 tsp black pepper
- ½ cup peanut butter
- 1 cup coconut milk
- One 15-oz can of chickpeas, rinsed and drained
- 2 cups chopped and frozen spinach

Throw it all in a pot and cook over high heat till it starts to bubble, typically around 10 minutes. Then turn it down and simmer for at least 30 minutes or until the sweet potatoes are soft and tender.

Also does great in a slow cooker, since the flavor complex of the curry, peanuts and coconut milk really get happier the longer they are allowed to play together.

Sesame Cauliflower

We love Asian food and were so happy when we modified this from Chocolate-Covered Katie *(chocolatecovered katie.com)*. We had it on brown rice, and it was delish! Serves 3 to 4, or just 2, if one of them is me.

- 1 head of cauliflower, chopped into florets
- 1/4 cup maple syrup
- 1/2 cup soy sauce or Tamari
- 1/4 cup rice vinegar
- 1 1/2 tsp roasted sesame oil
- 2 Tbsp minced garlic
- 1/2 tsp powdered ginger
- 1 1/2 Tbsp cornstarch or arrowroot
- 1/4 cup water
- sesame seeds and scallions, for garnish

Preheat oven to 450 degrees. Line baking sheet with parchment or silicone mat. Arrange cauliflower florets on pan and bake for 10 minutes. While it is baking, whisk together the wet ingredients, garlic, and ginger in a saucepan. Bring to a low boil. While waiting, stir together the cornstarch and water until the cornstarch is dissolved. Slowly whisk this into the mixture in the saucepan as soon as it boils. Turn heat to medium and cook 2 minutes, stirring frequently until it starts to thicken. Flip the cauliflower over and bake an additional 10 minutes. Add cauliflower to the sauce and stir until the cauliflower is covered. Serve over brown rice or your desired grain.

Side bar tip:
Why eat cauliflower? For one thing, just one serving (1 cup) provides 100 percent of your recommended daily Vitamin C intake! Also, it includes a quarter of your Vitamin K, which could help prevent mineral build-up in the arteries, a major risk factor for heart disease. Cauliflower has glucosinolates, which may help prevent cancer by protecting cells from damage and also have anti-inflammatory, antiviral and antibacterial effects. All good things!

Lentil Bolognese over Spaghetti or Spaghetti Squash

We were intrigued when we came across this yummy-looking recipe that uses fennel. I hadn't tried fennel before, but I was certainly willing to try it. Turns out fennel has a bit of a licorice flavor to it, and I'm not a fan of licorice. HOWEVER, when added to lentils and a host of other seasonings, the fennel brings about a satisfying meaty flavor. When you are vegan trying to do a Bolognese, this comes in handy! So here you go--a meat-free way to enjoy Bolognese sauce AND use fennel.

Serves 4

- 1 large (4 lb) spaghetti squash, halved lengthwise and seeded   OR 1 lb spaghetti noodles cooked as directed
- 4 cups vegetable broth
- 1 1/4 cup dried black (beluga) lentils
- 1/3 cup finely chopped fennel
- 1/2 cup finely chopped carrot
- 1 whole medium sweet onion, diced
- 1 cup red bell pepper, diced
- 6 garlic cloves, finely chopped
- 1 tsp fennel seeds
- 2 (15-oz) cans tomato sauce
- 1 tsp salt
- 1 tsp pepper, optional

To prepare the squash: If using the spaghetti squash, preheat oven to 350 degrees. Place squash halves side down on a baking sheet and roast for 40 to 45 minutes. Pierce the back of the squash to check to see if a knife can easily go through to see if it's done. Pull out of the oven and let cool cut side up for at least 20 minutes. With a spoon loosen the squash and scrape from the shell into a bowl.

To prepare the Bolognese: While squash or noodles are cooking prepare your sauce. Bring vegetable broth and lentils to a boil in a large saucepan over medium-high heat. Reduce to medium-low; stir once, simmer 25 minutes then drain.

In a large skillet over medium heat add fennel, carrot, onion, and bell pepper and cook until soft. Add a little water or extra vegetable broth to keep the vegetables from sticking. Add garlic and fennel seeds and cook stirring constantly for about 1 minute. Stir in tomato sauce and salt and pepper. Add the drained lentils, cover and cook over medium-low heat until mixture thickens, about 45 minutes. Remove the lid and stir occasionally.

Ingredients note: Black beluga lentils can be found easily on Amazon. Your grocery store may have them in cans. Goya is one popular brand.

Side bar tip:

Why would we want to use **fennel**?? For these awesome health benefits: it's a great source of potassium, Vitamin A, calcium, magnesium, Vitamin K, manganese, to name a few, a combination that adds up to better bone health and heart health, as well as lower blood pressure. The selenium in fennel appears to stimulate killer T-cells, which boost immune function! Who doesn't want that in the midst of a pandemic?

Brownie Fudge

My personal Go-To when I have to whip up something to take to a party. This is deceptively easy. The hardest part is remembering to make it ahead of time so it can come together in the freezer.

These are not merely another type of fudgy brownies. Rather, they straddle the line between pure chocolate fudge and a brownie. I tried this in a high-speed blender, but I found the food processor to be superior in terms both of the quality of the finished product and my frustration levels.

*adapted with much love and appreciation from Chef AJ

- 2 cups walnuts or pecans
- 3/4 cup cocoa powder
- 2 cups pitted dates
- 1 Tbsp vanilla extract
- 1 Tbsp maple syrup
- Sprinkle of salt

Pulverize the nuts in a food processor. Make sure to use the "S" blade, until they are the consistency of powder. Add the cocoa powder and crank it up again. Add the dates and hit it again until a ball forms. Then add the vanilla extract, maple syrup and salt and briefly process one more time until it is mixed well. Place in an 8 x 8 pan and freeze until firm, roughly two hours. Either use a silicone pan or line your pan with parchment paper, before dumping in, so that there will be no regrets later. Slice into squares and eat a few yourself before serving to others.

You may also use other nuts or nut combinations. This is very tasty, but very oily. I have to sop up the pool of oil that develops on top of the brownies like it's a pepperoni pizza and I'm on Weight Watchers again.

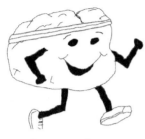

"Number one, like yourself. Number two, you have to eat healthy. And number three, you've got to squeeze your buns. That's my formula."

Richard Simmons

Exercise

I constantly try to get my patients to exercise. The benefits are tremendous, and it's never too late to start. Here's a partial list:

- Lower risk of:
  mortality whatever the cause
  cardiovascular disease (including heart disease and stroke)
  hypertension
  Type 2 diabetes
  adverse blood lipid profile
  cancers of the bladder, kidney, breast, lung, colon, endometrium, esophagus, and stomach
  falls (older adults)
  fall-related injuries (older adults).
- Reduced risk of:
  dementia (including Alzheimer's disease)
  anxiety
  depression
- Slowed or reduced weight gain
- Weight loss, particularly if combined with reduced calorie intake
- Prevention of weight gain following initial weight loss
- Improved
  cognition , sleep, physical function, bone health quality of life

[89] *(U.S. Department of Health and Human Services. Physical Activity Guidelines for Americans, 2nd edition. Washington, DC: U.S. Department of Health and Human Services; 2018.)*

We are concerned right now with the improving cognition and re-duced risk of dementia portions of that list. As we've already discussed, lowering your blood pressure and improving your diabetes both reduce your risk of dementia. And there are really exciting data coming out all the time about how exercise improves brain health.

They got better!

A 2010 study involving patients with Mild Cognitive Impairment had them perform aerobic exercise for 45 to 60 minutes a day, four days a week for six months. The control group was told to stretch for similar time periods. The good news? The exercise group improved their memory test scores! They got better! The control group, unfortunately but unsurprisingly, declined.[90] *(Laura D. Baker et al, 2010.)*

This was not a one-time finding. Numerous studies involving MRI scans of the brains of memory loss patients have shown aerobic exercise can reverse shrinkage in the hippocampus, the memory center of the brain. Bigger brain equals a better brain.

In another study, 120 subjects were randomized for exercise or no exercise. The exercise group walked for 40 minutes three times a week. At the end of a year, their MRI scans showed an increase in the volume of their hippocampus, which was nice. Still nicer, they showed improvement in their cognition as well. The control group had the typical decline that we all fear.[91] *(Kirk I. Erickson et al, 2011.)*

I could go on. There are more than 11,000 studies just since 2016 listed in the National Institutes of Health's online database discussing positive changes in patients' brain scans and actual brain function solely from using exercise as treatment.

How? Your new favorite word: neurogenesis. Neurogenesis simply means growing new brain cells. And that is precisely what we want to do. Previous dogma maintained that once you were an adult, you had all the brain cells you were ever going to get, so good luck. We now know this is not true. You can grow new brain cells and make new connections between existing cells. And exercise is a great way to make that happen.

This backs up what I tell my patients every day: Exercise has consistently been shown to be more effective than the pharmaceutical drugs at treating memory loss. And the side effects are way better too!

How?

Do we have to start training like an Olympic athlete to reap the benefits of neurogenesis? No. Most of the studies we mentioned above had their subjects ride a bike, walk on the treadmill or simply take a walk outside. I tell my patients all the time, I don't care what they do, only that they do it.

The magic appears to take place after you have been exercising about 45 minutes, most days of the week. That's when the brain gets flooded with happy hormones and fresh blood gets pumped way back into the deep nooks and crannies.

How much effort? Enough to get your heart rate up and get mildly sweaty. While you have to put some effort into what you are doing, the data do not point to any advantage from Herculean efforts as compared to moderate efforts.

What about strength training?

Multiple studies have shown that strength training does more than improve strength and antifragility.[92] *(Nicole C. L. Hess et al, 2017.)* We will include strength training as part of our exercise prescription. But what kind?

Again, we want our therapies to be effective and safe. Isometric exercises fit that description quite nicely. What are isometrics? Literally exercise without motion. Pushing with all your might against something that doesn't move. Think of pushing against a giant rock, or even holding yourself in the up position of a pushup. You are working hard, but barely moving.

Example: Put your hands together in front of your chest, right at heart level. As you take a slow breath in, start to push your hands together. Slowly build the tension for 10 seconds as you breathe in. Now, push your hands hard against each other, until they start to shake a bit while you exhale for 10 seconds. Now breathe normally while you slowly ease down on the tension for five seconds. Congratulations! You have completed your first upper body exercise for the day.

Isometric exercises were extremely popular in the 1950s and 1960s. They were (and still are) part of the Charles Atlas Dynamic Tension Course. I, myself, used dynamic tension and isometric exercises to rebuild my back after an injury in 2004. At that time, there was some concern about their effect on blood pressure, but this has since been proven false.[93] *(Paul G. Peters et al, 2006.)* [94] *(Broino Kiveloff et al, 1971.)* They have been proven to be safe and effective even for kids![95] *(David E. Fixler et al, 1979.)*

No Miracles, Just Hard Work

There have been many studies that showed promise for memory patients with just exercise alone.[96] *(Ashley Carvalho et al, 2014.)*

There have also been some good studies that showed no help whatsoever from exercise programs.[97] *(Sarah E. Lamb et al, 2018.)*

Dementia is a complicated, multi-faceted problem. That's why there isn't a single Silver Bullet solution. Consistently, the programs that produce the best results are the ones with multiple modes of treatment. That's why our memory protocol has four areas of focus, to help the whole body and mind begin to heal.

This happens quite often with my patients. They want to pick just the one part that looks easiest and do that one. While that is a great way to start, it's a lousy place to stop. The only way to enjoy the full benefit is to do the whole program.

The exercises:

"Train, don't strain" **Charles Atlas**

Although isometric exercises have been used for as long as people have been trying to develop their bodies, it was not until 1953 when German physiologists working on efficient ways to rehab debilitated patients started to heavily investigate isometric contractions. They found that contracting a muscle a little more than half of your perceived maximum effort for only six seconds, once a day was enough to create a 5 percent increase in strength in as little as one week![98] *(Th. Hettinger et al, 1953.)* Bob Hoffman, USA Olympic weightlifting coach from 1936 to 1968, also used isometrics as part of his arsenal in trying to build the world's strongest bodies.

The following exercises and routine are adapted from 1948 Olympic gold medal wrestling champion Henry Wittenberg's classic book on isometrics.

WARM UP PERIOD

You need a brief warm-up before you start isometrics. Marching in place for two to three minutes will suffice. If you feel up to it, then sit down and then stand up from a stable chair 10 to 15 times.

Heart rate up a little bit? A few beads of sweat feeling like they are making their way to the surface? Good. Time to move on.

ISOMETRIC PERIOD

The key to safely gaining strength through isometrics is the breathing. When in doubt, never hold your breath. At the beginning of each exercise, as you grasp your hands together and start to exert pressure, slowly start to inhale for 10 seconds as you gradually increase your force. Then start to exhale slowly through pursed lips

76

for another 10 to 12 seconds as you push or pull as hard as you can. A good barometer is push or pull until your hands are slightly shaking.

After this period of maximal effort, take another 10 seconds to ease the throttle down and start to relax your muscles gradually. Once you have finished relaxing, shake your hands out like you are trying to get water off them for a little bit. If you are out of breath, wait until you can talk normally before starting your next exercise. Taking your time and slowly building up tension and easing the tension off will go a long way toward both protecting and simultaneously strengthening your tendons and ligaments.

Remember, you only need to do each exercise once a day. The magic is in the consistent effort every day for the next few years. Your strength will increase every week, with all the benefits therewith.

PARADE REST

> **Start Position:** Stand up tall, feet hip-width apart, chest raised, stomach flat. Place your hands against the small of your back and grasp the right wrist with left hand.

> **Contraction:** Press the back of your hand against the small of your back. Increase pressure in your arms as if you are trying to pass your hands through your body as you inhale for 10 seconds. Press for 10 seconds as you slowly exhale and then ease off for 10 seconds. Shake your arms out, and once you are ready, move on.

PALM PUSH

> **Start Position:** Stand up tall, place palms of hands together in front of your chest, fingers pointing up. Forearms form a straight line in front of chest.

> **Contraction:** Inhale. Press your palms together, keeping forearms in a straight line. Hold maximal effort for 10 seconds, then start to relax for another 10 seconds. Shake your arms out. Once you're ready, move on.

BACK ARM PULL

Start Position: Stand or sit erect. Hook your fingers together in as strong a grip as is comfortable, straighten your arms as much as comfortable.

Contraction: Inhale. While keeping your arms stiff, try to pull them apart, and maintain your grip all through the maximal effort portion for 10 seconds. Ease off the tension and relax for 10 seconds. Shake your arms out. Once you can talk normally, move on.

OVERHEAD PULL

Start Position: Stand or sit erect. Join hands overhead in an interlocking grip.

Contraction: Inhale. Pull arms outward against your grip, building pressure for 10 seconds, then holding maximal contraction for 10 seconds while exhaling, then easing off the tension for another 10 seconds while you relax. Shake your arms out, and once you're ready, move on.

DEAD LIFT

Start Position: Use a loop of rope, or webbing for this next exercise. Honestly, I usually use the rope belt from my old terrycloth robe. Stand with both feet on top of the rope, inside the loop. You will be pulling on the rope, so make sure it is being securely held down with your feet. I find it more comfortable to put it right behind the balls of my feet. Grasp the rope in both hands, palms up. Assume a semi-squat position with your back straight, abs pulling your belly button into your spine to help protect your back. Take up slack in the rope by winding excess rope around your hands.

Contraction: Inhale slowly while using your legs and back and attempt to stand up straight against the resistance of the rope. Exhale slowly through the maximal contraction phase for 10 seconds, then start to ease off the pressure and relax for 10 seconds. Shake your arms and legs out, and once you're ready, move on.

CHAIR LIFT

Start Position: Sit up straight and tall in a stable, non-squishy chair, like a dining room table chair. Grasp the seat of the chair on both sides with your hands.

Contraction: Inhale. While holding fast to the chair, try to lift yourself and the chair using your legs. Chances are you won't be able to do it, but that is not the point. You are pushing up hard with your legs while pulling down with your upper body. Protect your back by squeezing your belly button into your spine. Exhale slowly through the maximal contraction phase for 10 seconds, then start to ease off the pressure and relax for 10 seconds. Shake your arms and legs out, and once you're ready, move on.

ANKLE PRESS

Start Position: Seated in your non-squishy chair, sit tall. Cross your ankles with right ankle beneath and pressing against your left ankle.

Contraction: Inhale. Force left foot back against right ankle while at the same time pushing your right foot forward against your left ankle. Protect your back by squeezing your belly button into your spine. Exhale slowly through the maximal contraction phase for 10 seconds, then start to ease off the pressure and relax for 10 seconds. Shake your legs out, once ready, move on.

Contraction: repeat the exercise as above, but this time place your left ankle beneath your right ankle.

BEHIND NECK PULL

Start Position: Sitting upright in your chair, place hands behind your head, right underneath that little bump on the back of your skull. (The occipital knob for you nerds out there.) Keep your elbows bent forward, fingers interlaced.

Contraction: Inhale. Push against back of your head with hands, while pushing against hands with the back of your head. Protect your back by squeezing your belly button into your spine. Don't go for broke on this one, you are not trying to rip your head off or strain your neck. Exhale slowly through the maximal contraction phase for 10 seconds, then start to ease off the pressure and relax for 10 seconds. Shake your arms out. Once ready, move on.

Stand up and smile, you have completed your basic strength exercises. You should feel pretty warm, maybe a little sweaty. You might feel tired the first day you perform this routine, but tired and exhausted is not the goal. This simple routine should feel like you are boosting your energy and saving it up. You should feel energized after you've completed it.

Remember, do each exercise only once a day. In order to get your prescribed 45 minutes of activity, you will need to take a walk, swim, ride an exercise bike or roller blade right after your isometrics. Do whatever you can safely most days of the week. If your schedule will not permit it, you could do your walk later in the day. But I recommend going ahead and getting it done now. I know if I wait and put something off till later, it's a great way to make sure I don't do it at all.

Stress

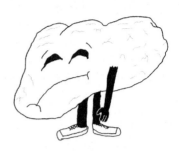

"Some days, doing 'the best we can' may still fall short of what we would like to be able to do, but life isn't perfect on any front--and doing what we can with what we have is the most we should expect of ourselves or anyone else." **Fred Rogers**

In my office, I see depression and anxiety in just about all my dementia patients. But which came first?

Overall, there is convincing evidence to support both the notion that early-life depression can act as a risk factor for later-life dementia, and that later-life depression can be seen as a pro-drome to dementia. ("Prodrome" is doctor-speak for an early sign or symptom of the onset of a disease.) There is also evidence to support the fact that these two kinds of depression show similar neurobiological changes, particularly white matter disease, either indicating shared risk factors or a shared pattern of neuronal damage.[99] *(Sophia Bennett et al, 2014.)*

A happy brain leads to a healthy brain. But it could also be that a healthy brain leads to a happy brain. So, which is it? No one is 100 percent sure yet. So, let's stick with what we do know. If we get our brain healthier, we will probably get a happier brain. And conversely, if we get our brain happier, we can get our brain healthier.

Later-life depression is associated with an increased risk for all-cause dementia, vascular dementia and Alzheimer's disease. The present research results suggest that it will be valuable to design clinical trials to investigate the effect of late-life depression prevention on risk of dementia, in particular vascular dementia and Alzheimer's disease.[100] *(Breno S. Diniz et al, 2013.)*

The problem certainly can be linked with both loss of neuronal function[101] *(Arash Salardini, 2019.)* and changes in the brain itself.[102] *(Thomas W. Meeks et al, 2006.)*

I describe it to my patients this way:

> Generic patient number three down the hallway used to have 30,000 neurons to control her emotions. (The true number is probably way bigger. But I'm bad at math, which is why I went into medicine.) Now she only has 30 neurons desperately trying to do the job of 30,000. It's an impossible job. And those little neurons will work until their batteries are completely empty. They can only be recharged by getting a good night's sleep.

This is what causes "sundowning," the phenomenon wherein patients exhibit dramatic changes in mental capabilities and emotional stability in the late afternoon/early evening. Tired neurons just run out of battery, and the emotions go wild.

That is the biological side, but then there is the deeper, more sinister side. Part of it is the horror of your situation. Imagine being handed the diagnosis of dementia. There is no hope; your future is gone. Your future consists of a slide into madness and loss of control.

To make matters worse, depression makes the symptoms of memory loss worse.[103] *(H. Gutzmann et al, 2015.)* The patient gets swept into a downward spiral as depression increases memory loss, and the increased memory loss increases depression, which increases the memory loss, which increases the depression, ad infinitum.

In our practice, we often get more bang for our buck by treating depression in patients rather than using the "memory pills" themselves.

Thus, the question is, how best to treat it?

Pushups Versus Pills for

Treating Depression

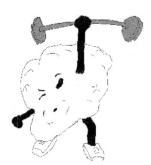

I started using exercise to relieve stress and treat my depressive symptoms in my late teens, early twenties. Exercise alone has been shown to work just as well as antidepressant medications for mild to moderate depression. Exercise can also be a potent addition that will improve depressive symptoms when it is used along with medications.[104] *(Peter J. Carek et al, 2011.)*

The data regarding treating anxiety symptoms with exercise are not quite so robust, but it remains true that exercise can still be quite helpful. It may even be effective in helping to treat various panic disorders.[105] *(Andreas Ströhle, 2009.)*

Exercise will kill two birds with one stone. As detailed in the previous sections, it can be a potent treatment for memory loss. Now we know it can also be a potent treatment for depression. Essentially, it is an excellent way of breaking that downward spiral we mentioned before. The exercise makes the depression better, which can make the symptoms of dementia better, which would make the depression better, which would. . . .Well, you get the idea.

Now, depressed people often don't feel like exercising. I get it. Using an antidepressant medication, even for a short time, can give you the motivation to get off the couch and do something positive for yourself. Or you could eat a baked potato.

An Apple a Day to Keep Depression Away

The Role of Diet

Vegetarians reported significantly less negative emotion than did omnivores in a 2010 study.[106] *(Bonnie L. Beezhold et al, 2010.)* The researchers followed up in 2012 with a randomized, controlled trial, and found that "Restricting meat, fish, and poultry improved some domains of short-term mood state in modern omnivores." [107] *(Bonnie L. Beezhold et al, 2012.)* One of their theories as to why this occurred has to do with the lower amount of arachidonic acid in vegetarian diets. Arachidonic acid is a pro-inflammatory compound, which they theorized could "adversely impact mental health via a cascade of neuroinflammation."

Neuroinflammation=Inflamed Brain. That's as bad as it sounds.

Remember, short-term inflammation around a wound is a good thing, but long-term it's quite bad for you. And that triples for your brain. An inflamed brain leads to lots of damage from the processes we have talked about previously: plumbing problems and oxidative stress. Again, the answer can be found in a big bowl of salad. Polyphenols from fruits and vegetables have been shown to reduce neuroinflammation.[108] *(Yousef Sawikr et al, 2017.)* A diet rich in polyphenols from the often-neglected produce department of your grocery store is being investigated as "a non-invasive, natural, and inexpensive therapeutic means to support a healthy brain." [109] *(Fernando Gomez-Pinilla et al, 2012.)*

A Gut Feeling

For me, the research around the gut microbiome is exciting. With an estimated 100 trillion different micro-organisms living and working in your intestines right now, the connection between what is called your "microbiome" and your brain is astounding. Scientists are learning more and more about it every day. You can easily fill a much larger and better-written book than this one dealing with this single subject. In a nutshell, what I tell my patients is that you have trillions of happy bacteria in your gut, and you want to keep them happy. And the only thing your happy gut bacteria eat is fiber. Period. Plants are your best, most easily digested, most easily enjoyed, most effective way to feed your gut bacteria and keep them happy.

Why do you want to keep them happy? My personal favorite reason is that 90 percent of your serotonin, dopamine, and other crucial hormones for mood and just plain old brain function are created in the gut! You go with your gut feelings, literally.

Happy hormones flowing around the brain make for a happy brain.

As I mentioned before, when we treat our dementia patients, we usually get much more bang for our buck treating their depression and anxiety than using memantine or donepezil. Why not allow your gut bacteria to replace the pills? More joy, fewer side effects.

Shut Up and Dance with Me:

Socialization to Treat Depression & Dementia

It is common for memory patients to avoid committing a social faux pas by isolating themselves. Indeed, feelings of loneliness are now thought to be a risk factor for dementia in older adults.[110] *(Tjalling Jan Holwerda et al, 2014.)* Isolation and a lack of social support have been linked to increased dementia risk.[111]
(Ross Penninkilampi et al, 2018.)

I admit this is another chicken vs egg debate. Does the isolation and lack of support lead to decline, or do people withdraw as the dementia sets in? The answer, of course, is "Yes."

Positive, supportive relationships have been proven to have an immensely beneficial effect on both physical and psychiatric health. The opposite, of course, is also true: social isolation increases certainty of depression/anxiety.[112] *(M. Sol Ibarra-Rovillard et al, 2011.)*

A 2014 study explored the power of our relationships on cognitive health. The researchers found "positive exchanges with friends and family were associated with less decline in perceptual speed, with these associations attenuated by adjustment for physical functioning and depressive symptoms. Negative exchanges with spouses were associated with poorer working memory performance."[113] *(Tim D. Windsor et al, 2014.)*

You will need a support group, a tribe, a team of people to gather around and help you through this. We love to think we are going to be John Wayne and pull ourselves up by our own bootstraps, but this problem is too big.

Navel Gazing for Dummies:

Meditation as Treatment for Depression/Dementia

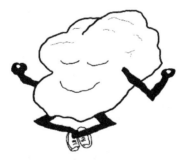

Why?

Meditation has shown positive effects in reducing physical and emotional symptoms such as psychological stress, depression, anxiety, fatigue, fear of recurrence and getting stuck in negative self-talk. That makes it an efficient strategy for coping with the disease and improving quality of life.[114] *(Raquel Vilanova Araujo et al, 2019.)* You can actually see changes in brain structure with meditation; it rewires the brain in as little as eight weeks![115] *(Rinske A. Gotink et al, 2016.)*

Also, it has been proven to be an effective therapy for major depression,[116] *(Madhuri R. Tolahunase et al, 2018.)* as well as for living with chronic pain.[117] *(Elizabeth F. Ball et al, 2017.)*

Mindfulness meditation has also been shown to help those with cognitive decline. A review of ten studies done in 2018 found a host of benefits from meditative practices, "including a reduction of cognitive decline, reduction in perceived stress, increase in quality of life, as well as increases in functional connectivity, percent volume brain change and cerebral blood flow in areas of the cortex."[118] *(Jesse Russell-Williams et al, 2018.)* An observational study in 2017 found similar improvements in cognition and function in patients with cognitive impairment.[119] *(Wee Ping Wong et al, 2017.)*

Remember, one of the ways to diagnose and distinguish the various forms of dementia is to take a look at an MRI scan and see what has been shrinking. These studies on meditation are exciting to me because instead of watching the brain atrophy, you get to watch it heal.

There is no medication I have found out there that can do that.

What?

What is Mindfulness meditation, and how do you do it? According to Wikipedia, "**Mindfulness** is the psychological process of purposely bringing one's attention to experiences occurring in the present moment without judgment."

Or as Jon Kabat-Zinn, the author of *Wherever You Go, There You Are*, puts it: "paying attention in a particular way: on purpose, in the present moment, and non-judgmentally."[120] *(Jon Kabat-Zinn, 1994.)*

How?

Find a quiet room, set a timer for five minutes, and concentrate on your breath going in and out of your lungs for the entire five minutes. Sounds simple, right? It's not. Immediately your mind starts to wander.

"Am I doing this right?"

"What did I have for lunch? What's for dinner?"

"Why did they have to have Kylo Ren's shirt off in *The Last Jedi?* "

"How many carrots can a baby bunny eat in one sitting?"

"Are crepes just pancakes with a better public relations campaign?"

This near constant chatter is very normal. It's just that we usually are too busy to notice it. Sometimes we are too busy on purpose as a way of avoiding certain thoughts or feelings. In those cases, meditation can be scary, because here you are sitting with nothing to distract you for five whole minutes. The magic trick of meditation is to notice the thoughts bumping around in your skull, but let them go by, returning your focus to your breath. That's it. It's the constant noticing you have been distracted, letting go of the distraction and getting back to the task at hand. The exercise is what trains your mind for The Real World.

One of the symptoms of chronic depression is the constant tape of negative thoughts looping over and over in your head often called "rumination." [121] *(Hui-Xia Zhou et al, 2020.)* And yes, that is the same word used to describe cows standing in a field chewing their cud. A depressed brain just keeps the same negative thoughts going over and over in the mind, like a hamster trapped on the wheel, just going around and around and around.

The brain training from a meditative practice helps to break that cycle. You recognize the same, stale old thought, and can let it go. It might come back, but you can start to release its grip on you. Over time, this can really make a big difference in your everyday life.

I do not recommend starting out with the chair and stopwatch technique. It's tough to get started, tough to keep going, tough to know if you are making any progress. Being depressed is tough enough; why make the cure difficult?

There are numerous books, videos, YouTube accounts to get you started, but I would highly recommend getting started the way I did: with an app for your phone or tablet. *HeadSpace, Calm,* or *10 percent Happier* are programs I've found to be immensely helpful dealing with my own depression and anxiety. Having been studied independently to verify they are effective at reducing stress and depressive symptoms, *HeadSpace* and *10 percent Happier* are designed to instruct you as you go, teaching you what your brain is doing and learning.[122] *(Elaine Yang et al, 2018.)* [123] *(Jennifer Huberty et al, 2019.)*

Get High on Your Own Supply:

Breathwork for Relieving Depressive Symptoms

What if you could just huff and puff and blow your depression away? For years, yoga practitioners have made such claims, and now modern science is starting to back them up. There is a growing body of evidence for using yoga breathing for the treatment of depression, anxiety, even post-traumatic stress disorders.[124] *(Richard P. Brown et al, 2009.)* A 2013 meta-analysis looking at using yoga to treat depression reported more favorable outcomes for yoga versus standard medical care, relaxation and even aerobic exercise.[125] *(Holger Cramer et al, 2013.)*

We are focusing on the breathing techniques; no chanting, no opening yourself up to any higher whatever. These are specific ways of breathing that provoke a specific physiological response. No belief required. Shaving your head is optional.

The type of breathing being studied isn't just breathing really fast till you pass out from hyperventilation. (Though that can be a fun party trick if you time it right.) No, they are specific breathing techniques with fun multi-syllable names such as ujjayi, bhastrika and Sudarshan Kriya. Patients start to experience relief of depression and anxiety in just 15 days using these breathing techniques, plus many notice improved cardiovascular function.[126] *(Edgar Toschi-Dias et al, 2017.)*

It is believed the techniques create a state of "calm alertness" by increasing "parasympathetic drive, calming of stress response systems, neuroendocrine release of hormones, and thalamic generators." In plainer English; subjects' brains plain-old worked better, therefore they felt better. Or maybe they felt better so their brains worked better? [127] *(Richard P. Brown et al, 2005.)* Either way, it's a non-pharmacologic treatment with very few side effects except for possible increased heart health. And this type of therapy has been shown to be more effective the longer you do it.[128] *(Lisa A. Uebelacker et al, 2017.)*

Getting started

BELLY BREATHING

The most basic technique is simply belly breathing. Take a full breath in but concentrate on your belly rising with the breath. Fill the lower parts of your lungs with air. Too many folks take very shallow breaths. You want to fill all the nooks and crannies with air. Now don't over inhale like you are about to jump into the deep end of the pool to find that quarter you dropped. Just take a deep breath, hold it for a half second, then let it all out. Then take another deep breath into your belly. If it helps you, put your hands on your stomach and concentrate on the sensation of your hands going up and down with the breath. Keep going till you feel better. That could be one minute, two, ten, whatever it takes.

Belly breathing is my personal Go-To Move when I'm feeling overwhelmed or anxious during the day. It usually takes about a minute or two, often less, of full belly expanding breathing, and my head is clear. It's especially useful as a way to hit my own personal reset button when I have to transition from seeing patients all day to getting home to spend time with my family. A few breaths in the car before walking in the door, and I'm a much better father and husband.

SQUARE BREATHING

Start breathing into your belly, like before. Start concentrating on your breathing, and on your next breath in, inhale to a count of four.

Now, hold your breath while counting to four.

Exhale while you count to four, and then hold with no breath in your lungs for another count of four.
Again, inhale to a slow count of four. Hold for a slow count of four. Exhale for a slow count of four and hold for a slow count of four. Repeat for at least 5 times, or as many times as you like.

The kids and I do this often as part of our bedtime routine. It is very relaxing. Do not do it while driving, or deep-sea diving.[129] *(Alina Prax, 2020.)*

THE WIM HOFF METHOD

Wim Hoff is a hero of mine, and while I find half of his writings to be the happy ranting of a mad man, I find the other half to be brilliant. He is a Dutch author, speaker and professional crazy man who has dedicated his life to studying how to expand the limits of human potential. He gained international fame for being The Ice Man, performing such feats of derring-do as:

- running a half-marathon above the Arctic Circle barefoot wearing only running shorts,

- swimming under the ice for more than 200 feet wearing only shorts, and

- summiting some of the highest mountains in the world wearing, you guessed it, just a pair of shorts.

He also has on multiple occasions stood for hours packed in ice while maintaining a normal internal body temperature. He routinely performs these stunts not just for attention, but for science. Multiple universities have studied Wim Hoff and his students.

The good news is you don't have to run out in the cold in your underwear. Like many others, I have found Wim Hoff's breathing techniques to be very beneficial for treating my own depression and anxiety.

This particular breathing technique is more technical and slightly more complicated than belly breathing or square breathing. You could stick to square breathing for years and be perfectly happy. But for those interested in a higher level, I offer this part of Wim's teaching.

1. While seated or lying down, take 30 or 40 full-belly breaths. Breathe fully into the belly and the chest, then let go, without force. Do not hold your breath like you do for square breathing.

2. When you get to your final breath, number 30 or 40, let the air out and hold it out for as long as you can without discomfort. You will be pleasantly surprised at how long you can hold your breath this way. Listen to your body; don't force anything. You are not trying to set any world records, just enjoy the relaxation.

3. When you feel the urge to breathe again, take a deep breath in and hold it for 15 to 20 seconds. Then release and relax.

4. Repeat the steps above two or three more times, paying attention to how you feel and adjusting your breath as needed.

5. Once you have finished your final round, let your breathing return to normal. Relax and enjoy the clear head and energy. Once you are ready, slowly get up and get on with your day.[130] *(Wim Hoff, 2020.)*

The whole thing should take around 20 to 25 minutes depending on how many breaths per round and how many rounds you do per session. There are several tutorials and walk-through videos online provided by Wim Hoff. That's what I do. Rather than trying to keep up with whether or not I'm on breath 19 or 22, I start a video and have Wim counting along with me on YouTube. Open YouTube, search for Wim Hoff breathing and several tutorials in multiple languages will pop up. If you are browser savvy, just type: https://youtu.be/tybOi4hjZFQ.

All of the above breathing techniques are very relaxing, and should always be done in a safe, comfortable place. I keep mentioning this, because I have heard too many stories of people doing the Wim Hoff method in a swimming pool and waking up underwater. Be smart, please.

Getting on the Couch:

Professional Help for Depression

Strategies outlined here will go a long way toward relieving depression and anxiety but may be insufficient for some patients. If you are one of those who have tried all of the above therapies and still need help, I recommend Cognitive Behavioral Therapy.

From the American Psychological Association website:

> Cognitive behavioral therapy (CBT) is a form of psychological treatment that has been demonstrated to be effective for a range of problems including depression, anxiety disorders, alcohol and drug use problems, marital problems, eating disorders and severe mental illness. Numerous research studies suggest that CBT leads to significant improvement in functioning and quality of life. In many studies, CBT has been demonstrated to be as effective as, or more effective than, other forms of psychological therapy or psychiatric medications.[131] *(No author cited, American Psychological Association, 2017.)*

It is important to emphasize that advances in CBT have been made on the basis of both research and clinical practice. Indeed, CBT is an approach for which there is ample scientific evidence that the methods that have been developed actually produce change. In this manner, CBT differs from many other forms of psychological treatment.

CBT is based on several core principles, including:
1. Psychological problems are based, in part, on faulty or unhelpful ways of thinking.

2. Psychological problems are based, in part, on learned patterns of unhelpful behavior.

3. People suffering from psychological problems can learn better ways of coping with them, thereby relieving their symptoms and becoming more effective in their lives.

CBT treatment usually involves efforts to change thinking patterns. These strategies might include:

- Learning to recognize one's distortions in thinking that are creating problems, and then to reevaluate them in light of reality.

- Gaining a better understanding of the behavior and motivation of others.

- Using problem-solving skills to cope with difficult situations.

- Learning to develop a greater sense of confidence is one's own abilities.

CBT treatment also usually involves efforts to change behavioral patterns. These strategies might include:

- Facing one's fears instead of avoiding them.

- Using role-playing to prepare for potentially problematic interactions with others.

- Learning to calm one's mind and relax one's body.

Not all CBT practitioners will use all these strategies. Rather, the psychologist and patient/client work together, in a collaborative fashion, to develop an understanding of the problem and a treatment strategy.

CBT places an emphasis on helping individuals learn to be their own therapists. Through exercises in the session as well as "homework" exercises, patients/clients are helped to develop coping skills, whereby they can learn to change their own thinking, problematic emotions and behavior.

CBT therapists emphasize what is going on in the person's current life, rather than what has led to their difficulties. A certain amount of information about one's history is needed, but the focus is primarily on moving forward in time to develop more effective ways of coping with life.

CBT has been shown to improve all manner of anxiety related disorders and has also been shown to help alleviate depressive symptoms even in patients with antidepressant medication resistant depression.[132] *(Antonia N. Kaczkurkin et al, 2015.)*

Numerous reviews have found that Internet-based therapy is just as effective as face-to- face therapy.[133] *(Gavin Andrews et al, 2015.)*

If all of that still doesn't work, well, maybe you do need a pill. Short-term use of a mood stabilizer/ antidepressant can be very helpful to ease the depressive symptoms enough to allow a patient to start one or more of the other therapies we have discussed here. The pill is a crutch so that you are better able to access all the other strategies to help ease your troubled mind. Don't think I'm knocking a crutch. Crutches are great when you have a broken leg. Use them when necessary.

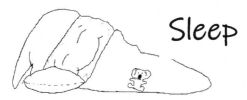

Sleep

Even though we all sleep, or at least need to, scientists who spend their lives studying sleep still don't completely understand it. Those of us in the health professions understand some of the benefits of getting enough sleep, and we are building a greater understanding of the detriments of sleep deprivation. So, in this section the focus will be on one of the biggest first world problems: not getting enough sleep.

We know that sleep deprivation is associated with high blood pressure, which increases your chances of heart attacks and stroke.[134] *(Sogol Javaheri et al, 2018.)* Lack of sleep also has been shown to affect memory and even the hippocampus of mice.[135] *(Robbert Havekes et al, 2016.)* Remember cramming all night for that exam the next morning? The lack of sleep meant your brain ended up trying to fight that exam with one arm tied behind its back. Your hippocampus was too tired to lay down any new memories. And to add insult to injury, your brain would likely be too tired it to readily retrieve the information it did have already in storage. That's definitely one thing I'll go back and tell myself when I build my time machine. That is if I can think clearly enough to use the time machine. Staying awake all night to build it might contribute to the buildup of amyloid plaques in the brain, a precursor to Alzheimer's.[136] *(Jae-Eun Kang et al, 2009.)*

A 2018 review article highlights changes in the brain down to the cellular and even DNA level derived from sleep issues.[137] *(Marie E. Gaine et al, 2018.)* Remember our old friend epigenetics? She's back, and she wants you to get more sleep, because not getting enough sleep is another way to damage your hippocampus. And a shrinking, unhappy hippocampus is one of the signs of Alzheimer's. The title of a meta-analysis also from 2018 sums it up nicely: "Sleep Disturbances Increase the Risk of Dementia." [138] *(Le Shi et al, 2018.)*

The best analogy I have heard compares the brain to a washing machine. You wouldn't want to remove your clothes halfway through the cycle, would you? That's how the brain feels without proper sleep--half clean, half done. In fact, that cleaning is one of the major reasons we sleep. It's just like your office building: that's when the cleaning crew arrives.[139] *(Philip G. Haydon, 2017.)*

Just Say No to Sleeping Pills

A review in the International *Journal of Psychiatry 2019* confirms what I found combing through the literature: Sleeping pills should not be the first choice, because they are not the best choice.[140] *(Scott Bragg et al, 2019.)*

Most over-the-counter sleep medications contain diphenhydramine, also known as Benadryl. Diphenhydramine is actually associated with confusion, and the American Geriatrics Society strongly recommends that patients over the age of 65 avoid taking it.[141] *(No author cited, 2019.)*

Benzodiazepines (such as Valium and Xanax) work short-term to calm a person but are generally not worth the long list of side effects—including death.[142] *(Anne M. Holbrook et al, 2000.)* Plus, the body adapts to the dose so quickly that after about two weeks you will need a bigger dose.[143] *(No author cited, 2008.)*

I do not prescribe Ambien, especially for older people. You might get to sleep, but you might also have the well-known, proven side effects of hallucinations, sleepwalking, sleep- driving, sleep-eating, and amnesia. Or you might just kill somebody.[144] *(Cheryl M. Paradis et al, 2012.)* There are better, cleaner ways of getting to sleep that have no side effects and no felony charges associated with them.

What about Melatonin?

The number of folks who use melatonin as a sleep aid (and not just on an airplane) has been growing for the past 20 years. Why not? Melatonin is a naturally occurring hormone produced by the body--more specifically, the pineal gland--to help the brain realize it's time for sleep. Supplementation with melatonin has been proven to be safe for months at a time, even in high doses.

But does it work? There's the rub. And the answer is. . .maybe.

Having reviewed a plethora of studies and articles, I have learned thatnthe scientific community appears to give a big old shrug when it comes to how effective melatonin can be. There are meta reviews saying it works well for everyone except those suffering from neurodegenerative diseases, like dementia. There are also studies showing no help at all for anyone. In my opinion, most of the study results that declare melatonin supplements work are pretty clouded by the possible intervention of the placebo effect, since the test subjects know they are taking melatonin in the trial. The double-blind randomized control trials either showed a slight benefit or none at all.

For folks suffering from neurodegenerative disease such as dementia or Parkinson's, proof that it helps is scant indeed. Which is unfortunate, since those are the folks who really need a good night's sleep.

So, should you take it? I'll give you the best answer science can give you right now: Maybe?

Beyond Counting Sheep, Cognitive Behavioral Therapy

So, you can't take pills for insomnia. What can we do?

Remember Cognitive Behavioral Therapy from the Stress section? It also works for insomnia.[145] *(Paul Sadler et al, 2018.)* A 2016 meta-analysis found that cognitive behavioral therapy works over the Internet just as well as it does when you sit face-to-face with a trained counselor.[146] *(Paul Sadler et al, 2018.)*

The year 2020 saw a proliferation of online counseling and tele-medicine options, e.g. BetterHelp.com or Try.talkspace.com.

Sleep hygiene is part of cognitive behavioral therapy.[147] *(Wee Ping Wong et al, 2017.)* What is sleep hygiene? Think of it as prepping the launch site. Just like my mom used to tell me, and now I tell my kids, straighten your room. Put away all the messy clothes, remove as much clutter as you can. Why? It relaxes your brain.

According to the CDC and the American Alliance for Healthy Sleep,[148] *(No author cited, 2016.)* here is a quick list of habits to start as soon as possible for a good night's sleep:

1. Keep a consistent sleep schedule. Get up at the same time every day, even on weekends or during vacations.
2. Set a bedtime that is early enough for you to get at least seven hours of sleep.
3. Don't go to bed unless you are sleepy.
4. If you don't fall asleep after 20 minutes, get out of bed.
5. Establish a relaxing bedtime routine.
6. Use your bed only for sleep and sex.
7. Make your bedroom quiet and relaxing. Keep the room at a comfortable, cool temperature.
8. Limit your exposure to bright light in the evenings.
9. Turn off your electronic devices at least 30 minutes before bedtime.
10. Don't eat a large meal before bedtime. If you are hungry at night, eat a light, healthy snack.

11. Exercise regularly and maintain a healthy diet.
12. Avoid consuming caffeine in the late afternoon or evening.
13. Avoid consuming alcohol before bedtime.
14. Reduce your fluid intake before bedtime.

These may sound overly simple, but all parents trying to get their babies down for the night know the power of a solid bedtime routine. It works for babies and children, and it works for adults.

Social Media Myths

An article being widely shared on social media about drinking a glass of water before bed to prevent a heart attack quotes the Mayo Clinic's Dr Virend Somers to increase its believability. And who doesn't want a super simple miracle cure to prevent heart attacks and stroke? It seems too good to be true. Which of course means that it is.

The Mayo Clinic and Dr. Somers have released a statement: "We have been informed of a recently circulated email regarding the use of aspirin, which included mention of Dr. Virend Somers and of Mayo Clinic. Neither Dr. Somers nor Mayo Clinic contributed to this email, which contains some information that is inaccurate and potentially harmful." [149] *(Shawn Bishop, 2010.)*

I searched through the Library of Congress listings to find any studies linking heart attacks and water before bed. This is the closest statement I could find: "Drinking water during the night can protect an increase in blood viscosity but there has been no evidence that drinking excessive amount of water prevents cerebral infarction. There was one report that the risk of myocardial infarction was lower in people drinking more than 5 glasses of water than those drinking less than 2." [150] *(Kikuo Okamura et al, 2005.)* In plainer English, if you are dehydrated your blood is thick and goopy, and that might make it easier to form a clot or blockage. If your blood is nice and hydrated, it can slide down your arteries smoothly and easily. But nowhere in the article does it mention drinking water as a magic cure for heart attacks.

The only thing drinking a big moose cup of water will prevent is a good night's sleep, since you will have to get up and go to the bathroom throughout the night. And interrupted sleep is linked to not only an increased in heart attacks, but also risk of death in general.

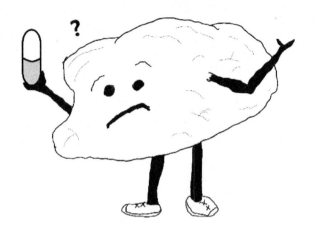

Supplements

Initially I was not going to put a supplements section in this book. I have way too many patients on various and sundry pills and potions who are still declining despite the gobs of money they shell out each month on supplements. It is akin to patching small holes on the roof while the foundation of the house cracks and splits due to the sinkhole underneath it. Patch the small holes once the underlying problems are addressed, then your patches will be far more effective.

Don't get me wrong, I love the promise of "All Natural" supplements that work better than pharmaceuticals. I take a handful of pills and a potion every day. The problem is most supplements simply do not work. Or I should say, they do not work enough. They are a small nudge of goodness that can be so easily overwhelmed.

Take diabetes medications as an example. We know standard diabetes medications do their job: they lower blood sugars. Give a non-diabetic person glipizide or even metformin and watch her or his blood sugar plummet to uncomfortable, probably even dangerous levels. But most of my diabetic patients out eat the effects of their diabetes pills and shots. One patient who stands out in my mind was in a health care facility, taking a hideous amount of insulin twice a day and with each meal. Nurses gave her the shots and handed her the pills, so it was not a case of noncompliance with the medical regimen. It was a noncompliant diet. She ate enough cookies, doughnuts, and crap to send her blood sugar over 500.

And so it is with supplements and their limited ability to effect massive change. You can toss buckets of water on a house fire all day long and be somewhat helpful. But if you never stop spraying gasoline into the inferno, what's the point?

Not a Complete Waste of Money

Another reason I was hesitant to include this section is that I feared I would be devoting too much time and space writing about all of the supplements that did not work. In this, I was happily surprised. There is cause for hope with some supplements. Again, I have to caution you. Even these supplements are just what the word implies, *supplemental* to a healthy diet, daily exercise and getting a good night's sleep. If you aren't working on the foundational pillars of the program, then you will receive little benefit from anything in this section. I will repeat, I have dementia patients right now taking many of the pills we are will go over, and they are still declining. Breaks my heart.

"Good Morning America" Test

If the cure for dementia in a single over-the-counter pill is truly discovered, you will not hear about it from an ad in the newspaper, tv commercial or pop-up in FaceBook. It will be all over the news, the subject of countless interviews, a topic for entire magazines, etc.

This list of over-the-counter supplements was compiled from different sales pitches, lectures, interviews and/or books on dementia. It is by no means comprehensive or exhaustive. It should cover most of what is recommended by reputable and non-reputable practitioners.

MAGNESIUM THREONATE

A 2018 review article found strong data to suggest a role for magnesium in migraine and depression, and emerging data to suggest a protective effect of magnesium for chronic pain, anxiety, and stroke.[151] *(Anna E. Kirkland et al, 2018.)* A 2019 cohort study that examined more than 20 years' worth of data from the Women's Health Initiative found that taking the daily recommended amount of magnesium was associated with a lower risk of developing dementia.[152] *(Kenneth Lo et al, 2019.)* However, a 2019 review article looking at magnesium supplementation confirmed magnesium supplementation increases the risk of rheumatoid arthritis and bipolar disease.[153] *(Wen-Wen Cheng et al, 2019.)*

So, what to do? Remember, when in doubt, eat food. Magnesium's RDA is 320mg for women and 420mg for men. Ladies can have 2oz of pumpkin seed kernels and be done for the day. A diet rich in seeds, nuts and beans will have plenty of magnesium in it. For the number nerds, run your diet through any of the free online diet calculators to see how your levels come out. If you are still low, then take a supplement. But remember, these are supplements to give you an edge in our fight against dementia. This section is practically worthless without the diet, without the exercise, without a good sleep routine.

COCONUT OIL

A quick Google search would have you believe that coconut oil has already cured Alzheimer's. A great deal of anecdotal evidence exists. But we're looking for facts, not sales hype. And coconut oil may be more hype than anything else. Coconut oil is a source of medium chain triglycerides (MCT), and there is evidence that MCTs could be beneficial for brain health. But a 2018 review article found that coconut oil consistently elevates LDL-C, the bad cholesterol linked to heart attacks and strokes. And "Even though coconut oil has relatively high MCT concentration, the clinical benefits of commercial MCT oils cannot be generalized to coconut oil."[154]

(Senthilkumar Sankararaman et al, 2019.) A review article from 2019 found coconuts were not even a good source of pure MCTs. The article also reported there is still not enough evidence to support the use of coconut oil for treating Alzheimer's disease.[155] *(Taylor C. Wallace, 2019.)* Conclusion: let's limit our consumption of coconut oils; there are better sources of the MCT oil out there. What good is it to take five greasy tablespoons of coconut oil a day if the only thing it will do is raise your risk of having a stroke and damage the very brain you are trying to protect? [156] *(Laurence Eyres et al, 2016.)*

MCT OILS

Data from clinical trials suggest use of MCTs can improve cognition in patients with mild to moderate AD, but only in patients who do not have "The Alzheimer's Gene," apoE4. This was initially seen as a barrier to the use of MCTs. But now we know that only 10 to 11 percent of all dementia patients are apoE4 positive. That leaves around 90 percent of patients who might benefit.[157] *(Alok Sharma et al, 2014.)*

So how do they work? Time to introduce you to Diabetes Type Three?[158] *(Mark A. Reger et al, 2004.)* The theory states demented brains are suffering from DM3 and starving all the time due to its insulin resistance. MCT oils are thought to produce ketones that the brain can use. Ketones are an alternative fuel source for the body, used during times of famine and lack. The demented, hungry brain can feast on these ketones and start limping toward a healthy state. Does it work? A Japanese study published in 2019 looked into short-term and long-term use of ketone therapy on patients with mild to moderate Alzheimer's disease. Patients were tested right after taking the supplements and the results showed no benefit versus a placebo. So no increase in cognition right after drinking the MCT oil. However, after taking the supplement daily for eight weeks, the study group started to show some improvement. And by week 12, they were doing even better.[159] *(Miho Ota et al, 2019.)* It's just like we said at the beginning: treatment of dementia is a long chess match.

These findings were confirmed in 2020 with a double-blind, randomized, placebo-controlled trial, using MCT oils this time. After

30 days, patients receiving MCT oil versus a placebo (canola oil) had improvement in their cognitive test scores.[160] *(Qing Xu et al, 2020.)*

So, it's a miracle, right? Well, not so fast. The patients in the 2020 study did have an improvement in their cognitive scores. On average, their score went up 2.62 points. The poor souls in the placebo group declined by 2.57. And neither group had any improvement in their ability to feed or dress themselves. We often use patient's ability to take care of themselves, feeding and dressing, as signposts for how far along a patient is in her/his disease. If I were an unscrupulous marketer, I would spin that study to show a 5.19 difference when using my product. That's not exactly how the math works. Yes, their test scores improved, but no impact on their daily lives was demonstrated.

The bottom line is, yes, MCT oils and Ketone supplements do offer some benefits. But their effect is mild to modest at best.

Omega 3/ PUFAs

Review articles from 2012,[161] *(Emma Sydenham et al, 2012.)*, 2016,[162] *(Marion Burckhardt et al, 2016.)* and 2018[163] *(Scheine Canhada et al, 2018.)* all failed to find any compelling evidence from hundreds of studies that treatment of dementia with Omega 3 (or PUFAs as they are sometimes called) makes any difference at all. OK, so once the damage is done, it's done. But what about prevention?

At best a diet rich in natural sources of Omega 3 can lower inflammation, and that is a good thing, and the whole plant-based diet that we recommend can get you all the Omega 3s you could ever want. Just eat a handful of walnuts daily.

"But I heard that the omega threes in walnuts are not as good as the fatty acids in fish."

First, we need to review the fact that fish is contaminated, so we don't want that anyway. And the type of Omega 3 fatty acids in walnuts, Alpha-linolenic acid (ALA), can be overwhelmed by Omega 6 fatty acids found in high amounts in the standard American diet. But guess what? You will not be eating the standard American diet, and you will not be overwhelming your system with pro-inflammatory Omega 6 fatty acids. So, toss back a handful of walnuts daily and skip the nasty fish burps from fish oil pills.

Allergic to nuts? There are vegan supplements out there made from algae and other aquatic plants. Fish don't make Omega 3 oils; they get them from their diet. So, skip the middleman/fish, and go to the source.

NRF2/ GLUTATHIONE

Nuclear factor erythroid-derived 2 related factor 2 (NRF2) is a well-studied transcription factor that activates the body's internal antioxidant mechanisms and detoxifying enzymes. Most neurodegenerative conditions such as Alzheimer's disease, Parkinson's disease, amyotrophic lateral sclerosis (or ALS, better-known as Lou Gehrig's Disease), frontotemporal dementia and Friedreich's ataxia are characterized by oxidative stress, misfolded protein aggregates, and chronic inflammation, the common targets of NRF2 therapeutic strategies.[164] *(Noemi Esteras et al, 2016.)* Interestingly, Alzheimer brains have fewer enzymes and pathways activated by NRF2 than do regular brains.[165] *(Kelsey E. Murphy et al, 2017.)* Activation of NRF2 pathways was shown to successfully "ameliorate deficits," at least in mice with Alzheimer's.[166] *(Gahee Bahn et al, 2019.)* In plainer English, it helped smooth over some of the problems the little demented mice were having.

Glutathione is an important antioxidant for the brain and has been considered a treatment target for a variety of neurological con-ditions. Your brain can make its own glutathione, or you can take a supplement. However, there is some debate as to whether or not oral supplements can cross the blood brain barrier.[167] *(R. Kannan et al, 1990.)* If that is the case, is there much use in taking oral glutathione supplements?

No, it becomes a source of false hope and waste of money.[168] *(Jörg B. Schulz et al, 2000.)* So, we are back to trying to activate it using the NRF2 pathway, so your body can create/use its own supply where it is needed. Circumin, resveratrol and sulfo-raphane have been shown to activate NRF2 pathways.[169] *(Angélica Saraí Jiménez-Osorio et al, 2015.)* A supplement called "Protandim" has also been shown to activate the NRF2 pathway,[170] *(Jamilah Abusarah et al, 2017.)* specifically those associated with the Alzheimer's pathway.[171] *(Brooks M. Hybertson et al, 2011.)*

CoQ10

Coenzyme Q10, also called "ubiquinol," is an enzyme involved with transporting electrons along the neurons, and also acts as an antioxidant. It has been studied as a potential therapeutic agent against neurodegenerative diseases for decades.[172] *(M. Flint Beal, 1999.)* But for years, no correlation was discovered. Numerous studies found no link whatsoever between CoQ10 and dementia, Parkinson's, ALS, etc. Finally, a study of 6000 Japanese men and women in 2014 found that low levels of CoQ10 were predictive of "disabling dementia." [173] *(Kazumasa Yamagishi et al, 2014.)* Does that mean we can treat existing neurological disease with CoQ10? The evidence is mixed at best. A double-blind, randomized, placebo-controlled trial in 2007 of CoQ10 using Parkinson's patients found no difference between the experimental and control groups.[174] *(Alexander Storch et al, 2007.))* In 2017, another gold standard double-blind, randomized, placebo-controlled trial that pitted CoQ10 against the particularly nasty form of dementia, Huntington's disease, again showed no difference between the experimental groups.[175] *(Andrew McGarry et al, 2017.)*

A study published in 2018 found that rats engineered to have Alzheimer's fared better than the control group with less harmful remodeling of the hippocampus and fewer plaques in their brain if they were fed a diet loaded with Kenaka powder (a version of Ubiquinol) with Vitamin C.[176] *(Javier Frontiñán-Rubio et al, 2018.)* A 2019 study in which mice were "artificially aged" by giving them mega doses of galactose, the sugar found in milk, plus laser surgery to mimic atherosclerotic blockages reported that CoQ10 with and without infrared light therapy did report benefits in memory in various trials. However, there was no control group, and the whole method of aging mice using galactose is somewhat controversial. It's another small piece of evidence for CoQ10, but it's not a game changer.[177] *(Farzad Salehpour et al, 2019.)*

CoQ10 in its various forms does appear to be very safe, and helpful in dealing with heart disease. [178] *(Abhinav Sharma et al, 2016.)* The evidence for using it to treat and prevent dementia is less than compelling. If you want to take it for the heart benefits, please be my guest.

But what if you could just make your own?

Remember, ubiquinol is an antioxidant. When it takes out a free radical, it needs to be recharged. Researchers exposed spent ubiquinol, called "ubiquinone," and dietary chlorophyll to the kind of light that reaches our bloodstream, and it was recharged back into battle-ready ubiquinol. The researchers further theorized that this combination of sunlight and chlorophyll from green leafy vegetables would not only increase antioxidants in the body, but also contribute directly to ATP synthesis in the mitochondria. As they concluded "consumption of plant chlorophyll pigments, animals, too, are able to derive energy directly from sunlight." [179] *(Chen Xu et al, 2014.)*

ASHWAGANDHA

Ashwagandha is an herb that has been used in Indian Ayurvedic medicine for hundreds of years. Review articles from 2010[180] *(M. R. Ven Murphy et al, 2010.)* and 2011[181] *(Narendra Singh et al, 2011.)* sound like they were written by The Committee to Promote Ashwagandha, if there were such a thing. (A quick Google search produced no hits as of this writing.) In Ayurvedic medicine, Ashwagandha is called a "rasayana," an elixir used to "increase human health and longevity." It is considered an adaptogen, a nontoxic medication that normalizes bodily functions that have been disrupted by chronic stress, through correction of imbalances in the neuroendocrine and immune systems. As for the brain, the review articles point toward numerous studies in which Ashwagandha slows, stops, reverses or removes neuron atrophy and synaptic loss, at least in petri dishes and lab mice.

That sounds good in theory, but what about the actual clinical trials in humans? In 2017 there was a randomized, double-blind, placebo-controlled trial of 50 adults with mild cognitive impairment. After eight weeks, the ashwagandha group "demonstrated significant improvements compared with the placebo group in both immediate and general memory" on a wide variety of tests.[182] *(Dnyanraj Choudhary et al, 2017.)*

Another review article from 2020 does back up the claims of "neuroprotective properties" for ashwagandha, but at the same time admits that most of the data are from preclinical trials with only a handful of actual clinical trials.

How does it protect the brain? It somehow gets the mitochondria (Recall your 8th grade biology: mitochondria are the powerhouses for the cells.) firing properly, while helping the inner lining of the arteries, the endothelium, to function again. It also appears to help clean out old, malfunctioning cells through apoptosis (which is defined as the death of cells that is part of an organism's normal growth and development).[183] *(Nawab John Dar et al, 2020.)* Finally, ashwagandha helps to turn on our internal anti-inflammation and oxidative stress mechanisms. I agree with another review article published in 2020: Ashwaghandha appears to have a good amount of neuro-protective potential in various brain disorders, though our understanding of how it works is still vague at best.[184] *(Sultan Zahiruddin et al, 2020.)*

BACOPA

Bacopa is a perennial creeping herb long used in Ayurvedic medicine to improve cognition and reduce depression and anxiety. Bacopa has been well studied, and most of the data are encouraging. A meta-analysis from 2014 reviewed several randomized, placebo-controlled trials and concluded Bacopa given for at least three months does improve cognition.[185] *(Chuenjid Kongkeaw et al, 2014.)*

A study I particularly like is a randomized double-blind placebo- and active-controlled clinical trial published in 2014 comparing an herbal blend including bacopa to placebos and also to the leading Alzheimer's drug, donepezil. After three months, the herbal blend group not only showed improvement over the placebo group, but also beat out the donepezil group. While exciting to me, it's not surprising, since as we discussed earlier, donepezil can only slow down the symptoms of the disease. In this study, the herbal preparation group showed significant improvements in inflammation and oxidative stress, which was theorized to be the main mechanism of improvement. [186] *(Ananya Sadhu et al, 2014.)*

POLYPHENOLS

Oxidative stress, mitochondrial dysfunction and rampant inflammation are commonly found in brains of dementia patients.[187] *(Jintang Wang et al, 2018.)* "While mitochondrial dys-function could cause neuroinflammation, neuroinflammation could also cause mitochondrial dysfunction."[188] *(Heather M. Wilkins et al, 2016.)*

The easiest way to describe oxidative stress is basically as cellular rust. It's much the same chemical reaction, whether it be an iron bar or your brain. A rogue destabilized oxygen molecule flies through your body stealing electrons from other atoms until it's satisfied. Of course, this destabilizes the neighborhood, creating more rogue oxygen atoms (officially called "Reactive Oxygen Species"), which attack their neighbors who attack their neighbors, much like your common zombie apocalypse. This is troublesome for your boat; but in your brain, it's disastrous.

There is hope. Polyphenols are strong antioxidants, proven to work both in human and animal trials. Regular consumption of dietary polyphenols is proven to inhibit reactive oxygen species (ROS) and proinflammatory cytokines, as well as improve mitochondrial function. Again, these processes are believed to be the root of neurodegenerative disorders such as Alzheimer's, Parkinson's disease, and stroke. A 13-year-long clinical study "indicated that a higher intake of these antioxidant polyphenols helps improve memory and has the potential to inhibit brain aging."[189] *(Jintang Wang et al, 2016.)* The antioxidants also decreased homocysteine, a brain toxin we will discuss later in the B12 section, which contributes to the pathology of neurodegenerative diseases.[190] *(Rita Moretti et al, 2019.)*

110

So, of course, now you want to know where to get poly-phenols. Glad you asked. Polyphenols, also called "flavonoids," are readily found in fruits, such as apples, pears, apricots, cherries, berries, and grapes. Vegetables, such as carrots, tomatoes, onions, garlic, cabbage, and celery can contain up to 200–300 mg of polyphenols.[191] *(Hassan Rasouli et al, 2017.)*

Well-studied flavonoid compounds found in supplements are curcumin, resveratrol, quercetin, which have all been found to have amazing abilities to reduce inflammation, improve mitochondrial health, and heal the blood brain barrier, as well as improve gut health in a way to improve communication to the brain.[192] *(Jintang Wang et al, 2018.)* More than one study pushed the idea that these compounds should be considered as a replacement for the standard pharmaceutical treatment for dementia.[193] *(Syed-Badrul Syarifah-Noratiqah et al, 2018.)* Who can argue with that: fewer side effects and they attack some of the root causes of brain deterioration. We definitely recommend getting polyphenols in a pill, but also in their original packaging, fruits and vegetables.

TAURINE

Grab a can of energy drink from the nearest teenager, read the ingredient list, and you'll find taurine. Taurine is a non-essential amino acid with antioxidant properties. It is used in energy drinks mostly due to the idea that it can improve athletic performance.[194] *(Thomas G. Balshaw et al, 2013.)*

A 2017 review article detailed numerous neuroprotective effects, especially when combined with caffeine. Unfortunately, the bulk of the data came from essentially poisoned lab rodents. The rat or guinea pig given a neurotoxin fared better when given taurine versus the control animal. The researchers note that aged or damaged human brains have lower taurine levels than normal, healthy brains. It's not much of a jump to say that taurine could be helpful in those cases.[195] *(Christine Perdan Curran et al, 2017.)*

An interesting side note, while caffeine and taurine could be healthy for older brains, the opposite appears to be true for young, adolescent brains. It appears it may be best to only let energy drinks give your grandpa wings, not your nephew.

L-CARNITINE

L-carnitine has been well studied for its ability to improve mitochondria function. The studies range from three months to one year, with L-carnitine dosage ranging from 1.5 to 3 grams per day. The trials reported benefits of L-carnitine over placebo in patients with mild cognitive impairment or suspected Alzheimer's disease. Unfortunately, for patients a bit further along in their disease process the results were "less conclusive." This points toward a "therapeutic window," but more studies would need to be done to establish the optimal timing. Still, in terms of prevention, I always think Right Now is a great time. "Additional studies and reviews showed that [L-carnitine] can slow pathologic decline in young patients with AD, improve clinical features of AD, and, when administered as a component of a vitamin formula, can delay cognitive decline in both early- and late-stage AD." [196] *(Gregory E. Bigford et al, 2014.)*

While red meat is the greatest source of L-carnitine, consumption of red meat is associated with significant decline in cognition.[197] *(Emiliano Albanese et al, 2009.)*,[198] *(Paul Giem et al, 1992.)* A 2020 review paper confirmed that supplementation with one gram of L-carnitine two or three times a day does im-prove cognition in a variety of studies and is well tolerated. More is not better though. Doses higher than three grams daily did not appear to offer greater benefit, and your intestines can't absorb anything greater than two grams at a time.[199] *(Alina Kepka et al, 2020.)*

GINKGO BILOBA

Ginkgo Biloba is an ancient tree, with fossils dating back 270 million years. Native to China and revered in Japanese culture, it has been used as medicine as far back as the 15th century. It has been very well studied, with mixed results. There is currently no evidence that Ginkgo can prevent Alzheimer's disease or other forms of dementia.[200] *(Steven T. DeKosky et al, 2008.)* [201] *(Thammanard Charemboon et al, 2015.)* [202] *(Mengmeneg Yang et al, 2014.)* However, for the folks who already have dementia, it does appear to be helpful. A meta-analysis of randomized placebo-controlled trials in 2018 determined supplementation with ginkgo for 22 to 24 weeks did help alleviate "behavioral and psychological symptoms of dementia." Symptoms such as agitation, anxiety, depression, disinhibition all improved with ginkgo in the different trials.

Again, looking at the data, a statistically different improvement and real-world difference are not the same. I like this comparison of different studies because it does measure caregiver distress, which also improved when the patient was given ginkgo. Admittedly, sometimes the difference between the two groups was small. The composite scores indicate depression on gingko was 1.93, on placebo 2.00. OK, so yes, folks were helped with ginkgo, but not cured.[203] *(Egemen Savaskan et al, 2018.)*

Other review articles also found that treatment with ginkgo biloba 240 mg for around 24 months appears to be quite safe and at least mildly beneficial in both cognition and behavioral symptoms. So, I think it is well worth a try if you or someone you love is dealing with dementia. It's in the category of probably not going to hurt you, and it might even help. All the studies indicate doses less than 240 mg per day are ineffective, and any time frame less than 24 weeks also ineffective.[204] *(Serge Gauthier et al, 2014.)* [205] *(Rainer Spiegel et al, 2018.)* [206] *(Meng-Shan Tan et al, 2015.)*

GABA

Mixed reviews. There is a good deal of evidence that GABA as a supplement cannot pass the blood brain barrier. Even studies that tout a positive effect admit that the results are mild,[207] *(Ken Kihara et al, 2016.)* and often not statistically significant.[208] *(Anna Leonte et al, 2018.)*

A 2015 review paper heavily suggested that most of the anec-dotal evidence toward GABA supplementation can be linked to the placebo effect.[209] *(Evert Boonstra et al, 2015.)*

> **Anecdote:** When I worked in the prison infirmary, some of the older nurses there would talk about the good old days when they gave inmates "The Blue Pill" for their pain. For really, really bad pain, the nurses could switch to "The Red Pill." And if the inmate were sick, they administered "The Green Pill." The pills were all sugar pills, but the nurses swore up and down that they worked great. Much better than the acetaminophen or ibuprofen we were currently giving them. So never completely discount the placebo effect. It can be really powerful.

The only real positive feedback appears to be that GABA as a food supplement may influence gut flora activity, which could in turn provide an indirect action on the brain. Now, that is not a bad thing, so don't count GABA out yet as a potential contender. However, there is an abundance of evidence that a plant-based diet supercharges your gut flora in a way that can help depression, anxiety, insomnia, and cognition already. So GABA supplementation may not be needed.

VITAMIN B12, B COMPLEX VITAMINS, FOLATE

Homocysteine is an amino acid common in the body, derived mostly from eating meat.[210] *(WebMD www.webmd.com/heart-disease/guide /homocysteine-risk#:~:text.2020)* (It is linked to heart disease and stroke. An elevated reading is usually because of a deficiency in vitamins B12, B6 or folate (another B vitamin).[211] *(Arturo J. Martí-Carvajal, 2017.)*

High homocysteine levels are bad for the heart, but what about the brain? A 2011 meta-analysis of 8,669 patients established a link between elevated homocysteine and the incidence of dementia. While the researchers were careful not to suggest cause and effect, they did go on record as saying treatment with B12 and folate could net a 20 percent reduction in risk of dementia.[212] *(David S. Wald et al, 2011.)* But the exact same year, the German Medical Association released a review paper that found no benefit in cognitive status in any of the randomized placebo-controlled trials they studied.[213] *(Thorleif Etgen et al, 2011.)*

So, which is it? A 2015 review article did back up the idea that high homocysteine levels and low levels of B vitamins could be a risk factor for developing Alzheimer's disease.[214] *(Liang Shen et al, 2015.)* Another review in 2017 concluded high homocysteine levels were linked to increased risk of cognition impairment in patients with Parkinson's disease.[215] *(Yi Xie et al, 2017.)* But again, other studies find no benefit from treating the patients already suffering from memory loss.[216] *(Anne Ws Rutjes et al, 2018.)* [217] *(Andrew H. Ford et al, 2012.)*

I take B12 for my depression and anxiety, and it has made a big difference. I continue to take it to help prevent dementia. But unfortunately, my personal experience with treating patients with B12, whether it be high-dose injections or simple over the counter pills backs up the idea that once the disease takes hold, it's of little value.

If you go back to the beginning of this section, you read that homocysteine is an amino acid associated with low B vitamins, but also with eating meat. Perhaps researchers are missing the boat. Supplementing with B vitamins does not appear to have much difference in heart disease, despite the link between homocysteine and heart disease.[218] *(Arturo J. Martí-Carvajal et al, 2017.)* But we already know, and have already proven, a whole plant food diet reverses heart disease by removing from the diet the main source of homocysteine--animal products.[219] *(Caldwell B. Esselstyn, Jr., 2016.)* So we cycle back to the diet section. It's the food.

VITAMIN D

It is estimated that more than 1 billion people worldwide are Vitamin D deficient.[220] *(Michael F. Holick, 2007.)* The elderly have it even worse. Some causes are as simple as not going outside enough, and others as complicated as the internal vitamin D processes break down as we get older. [221] *(Michael F Holick et al, 1989.)* Vitamin D deficiency has been linked to many age-related diseases, like Alzheimer's disease and other various inflammatory conditions.[222]

115

(A. Pines, 2014.) Mice and rats treated with vitamin D show a protective effect against physiological processes that lead to dementia.[223] *(Véréna Landel et al, 2016.)* A 2019 meta-analysis found higher levels of vitamin D in the blood was associated with lower risk of developing Alzheimer's in humans.[224] *(Ahmad Jayedi et al, 2019.)* However, a 2020 review article confirmed what I had already been reading, and what I see in my practice--treating patients already sick with vitamin D gives you mixed results, at best.[225] *(Sadia Sultan et al, 2020.)*

In my practice, many of my patients feel better and have more energy when their vitamin D levels rise with supplementation, as I, myself, do. My vitamin D levels were 19, way below normal. I noticed a big difference after a few months popping those little golden pills. Unfortunately, my dementia patients do not get their memories back when we get their levels back to reach normal. My guess is there must be a therapeutic window, a sweet spot where you get your levels up to normal before the damage gets so severe it's noticeable. I do recommend vitamin D3 4000 units daily to safely get levels above 50 nanograms per milliliter, which is the measure most labs use. [226]*(Véréna Landel et al, 2016.)* And you should have started taking it yesterday, for best effect.

VITAMIN E

A few decades ago, vitamin E was being hyped as the cure for heart disease and cancer, until a 2005 meta-analysis linked high-dose vitamin E supplementation (400 IU daily) with an increase in all-cause mortality and therefore "should be avoided."[227] *(Edgar R. Miller 3rd et al, 2005.)* Many other researchers jumped on the bandwagon, and Vitamin E was as good as dead. The current thinking on that has been reversed, thankfully.[228] *(Erin L. Abner et al, 2011.)* Now that we are reasonably certain it's not going to kill you, is it going to help you?[229] *(Andrea J. Curtis et al, 2014.)* Yes, but only when taken naturally. Different meta-analysis and review articles have shown that taking a vitamin E supplement can be really helpful for rats artificially given dementia.[230] *(Agnese Gugliandolo et al, 2017.)* [231] *(Mehrdad Jahanshahi et al, 2020.)* Unfortunately it has little to no effect on humans suffering from mild cognitive impairment or Alzheimer's disease,[232] *(Declan Browne et al, 2019.)* [233] *(Richard J. Kryscio et al, 2017.)* [234] *(Nicolas Farina et al, 2017.)* the only exception being when you eat a diet naturally rich in vitamins and minerals, like we recommend. [235] *(Dagfinn Aune et al, 2018.)*

HERSHEYS VERSUS FLINTSTONES

Who wouldn't want to hear that chocolate can help prevent dementia! That is exactly the sort of research partly being funded by the Mars Corporation. Yes, the maker of M&Ms is looking into the health benefits of cocoa extracts. Back in 2015 there was a study[236] *(Daniela Mastroiacovo et al, 2015.)* to see if patients tested better on three different cognitive tests after drinking cocoa drinks of various potencies for 8 weeks. The subjects drinking the highest amount of cocoa flavonols had the highest mild improvements in test scores. A larger follow up study in 2021 found similar benefits.[237] *(Richard P. Sloan et al, 2021.)* So, it's time to start knocking back the Yoo-hoos, right?

Not so fast. The 2021 study pointed out that it could just be the increased nutrition from flavonols in general. Remember our discussion of polyphenols a few pages ago? Flavonols, or flavonoids, are just another name for the antioxidant compounds found in all foods. Plants have the most, processed junk foods and steak have the least amount. And what do most Americans eat? The least nutritious foods on the planet, correct. As the authors of the flavonol study said, "the general US public has a poorer diet quality than the bottom tertile of participants in this study and may thus tenably experience cognitive benefits from increasing their diet quality and flavonol intake."[238] *(Richard P. Sloan et al, 2021.)* In plainer English, most folks eat so incredibly poorly that even a small increase in anything healthy can help their poor suffering brains out at least a little bit.

And don't unscrew the top of that Yoo-hoo bottle just yet. The first reported results from the COSMOS-Mind trial show no benefit over placebo from cocoa flavonol supplementation. What did help? A simple multivitamin. "Daily multivitamin-mineral supplementation appears to slow cognitive aging by 60% or by 1.8 years," according to study author Dr. Laura Baker. [239] *(Pauline Anderson, 2021.)*

No miracle pills

I'm sure some of you reading this book are asking, "yeah, but what about Compound X I just read about on that ad on FaceBook?" As I said at the beginning of this chapter, this is not nor can it be a comprehensive list of every supplement ever produced everywhere. That book would be immense, and totally out of date as soon as it was published.

Take a look at the few substances in this chapter that have been shown to improve a few test scores in a couple of studies: multi-vitamins, a few other vitamins, polyphenols like turmeric/curcumin, resveratrol and bacopa. All the active helpful compounds found in those supplements are derived from plants. Remember, it's the food. Your food, your daily diet is the main source of polyphenols, vitamins, all of it. These other pills and potions are to be supplemental to the main thing, a plant heavy diet.

Enlisting Help

My design and dream for this book have been essentially to outline a DIY program anyone can start Day One. The research we have gone over shows that the *Keep Your Marbles* program will protect your brain from most of the causes of dementia. There are a handful of helpful pharmaceutical strategies often recommended by lifestyle medicine and functional medicine practitioners. We will briefly discuss them here, but really if you are interested further you will have to schedule an appointment with a medical practitioner with experience handling such matters.

HORMONE REPLACEMENT THERAPY

Often touted as a cure for many ills and a strong treatment for dementia, hormone replacement therapy has been widely studied. As with so much in dementia treatment, it's a mixed bag at best. The Women's Health Initiative Memory Study, a gigantic multi-center, randomized, double-blind, placebo-controlled trial involving more than 7,000 women found that not only does hormone replacement therapy not protect against dementia, it actually raises the risk of dementia and cognitive decline.[240] *(Michael C. Craig et al, 2005.)* A 2018 review found similar results, increased risk of dementia but also increased risk of "coronary events, venous thromboembolism, breast cancer, gallbladder disease, and death from lung cancer." [241] *(Patricia Van Leer, 2018.)*

So why keep trying? There are some arguments for a "therapeutic window."[242] *(Pauline M. Maki et al, 2012.)* Starting the hormone replacement therapy much earlier, right around the time of menopause, may grant women some protection against Alzheimer's, or at least have no negative impact.[243] *(Victor Henderson et al, 2005.)* A study out in 2011 supports that point of view, and specifies that starting the hormones later in life, around 76 years old, "could have deleterious results." [244] *(Rachel A. Whitmer et al, 2011.)*

What do we do with this? Should we avoid hormone replacement therapy? I often talk with my patients about risks versus benefits for whatever pills or treatments they are about to start. There are risks associated with any and all treatments for anything. Yes, there are risks with hormone replacement therapy: increased risks of breast cancer and heart attacks, on top of starting too late and increasing the risk of dementia. But how big a risk? If the risks discovered in the Women's Health study were "extrapolated to postmenopausal women aged 50 to 59 years, the absolute risk of dementia from standard dose hormone therapy would be rare, representing about one additional case among 1000 women using hormone therapy for five years."[245] *(Pauline M. Maki et al, 2012.)* Sounds great, unless you or your grandma are the lucky number out of 1000.

Clearly, considering risks versus benefits, I cannot recommend taking hormone replacement therapy solely for brain protection. However, if you start earlier enough in life to treat symptoms due to menopause (and there are many), just be aware of the risks when you make that decision. And be sure you are working with a doctor with a good pedigree and a long track record of following and supporting patients who use hormone replacement therapy.

ANTIVIRALS

For me, the viral theory for the cause of Alzheimer's disease is the scariest. Get a cold sore, get dementia. Dr. Alzheimer and the other early pioneers in dementia medicine theorized an infectious cause for the disease.[246] *(A. Alzheimer, 1911.)* We now know there is indeed a link between dementia and different viruses, such as Herpes Simplex 1, [247] *(Vincent Chin-Hung Chen et al, 2018.)* and other brain-loving bacteria like chlamydia, and the family of bacteria called "spirochetes."[248] *(Ghulam M. Ashraf et al, 2019.)* Spirochetes, if you remember from your 8th grade biology, are the bacteria with flagella running and twisting along the sides. They cause diseases such as Lyme disease, syphilis and relapsing fever among other things on my list of Things Not to Get.

How does it work? The idea is inflammation from the infections becomes chronic, leading to the creation of the famous protein tangles and mitochondrial dysfunctions that ultimately lead to dementia. [249] *(James Stefaniak et al, 2016.)*

What do we do about it? A review article in 2018 studied the records of more than 30,000 Taiwanese patients, finding not only a link between HSV-1 and dementia, but that treating herpes with antiviral medications actually reduced patients' risk of developing dementia.[250] *(Nian-Sheng Tzeng et al, 2018.)* Does that mean we should all rush out to pop some antiviral meds if we have ever had a cold sore? The viral theory itself, let along treating dementia patients with antivirals, is still very much unproven.[251] *(Avindra Nath, 2018.)* [252] *(Avindra Nath, 2019.)* A similar review article in 2019 investigated the nationwide records of 7,000 patients over 11 years and failed to find any correlation between HSV and dementia.[253] *(M. Torniainen-Holm et al, 2019.)*

I have tested a handful of my own dementia patients, and they usually have some level of viral load, some quite high. I have treated them with various antiviral medications, because there might be some benefit. I must warn you, none of them had sudden reversal of his or her disease. Again, it might be another hole in the roof that we could patch. It also might be a waste of time. [254] *(Ruth F. Itzhaki, 2016.)* Talk to a clinician with experience in such matters for more details.

MOLD

If the idea of viruses chewing up your brain isn't scary enough, there is also evidence of fungal colonies in Alzheimer's brains.[255] *(Ruth Alonso et al, 2014.)* This is a debated topic, but a study in 2017 found evidence of chronic infections of both bacteria and fungi in brains of Alzheimer's patients.[256] *(Diana Pisa et al, 2017.)* It appears that the fungal and bacterial infections/colonizations are present all through the life cycle, in young brains as well as old, but the percentages are higher in Alzheimer's brains.[257] *(Ruth Alonso et al, 2018.)* Why is that? Is it the fungal infections making the patient sick, or is it that a sick patient that cannot fight off the infections? [258] *(Róisín M. McManus et al, 2017.)* No one is sure. It is known that Alzheimer's brains have a leaky blood brain barrier, which may be letting the pathogens into the brain.[259] (Róisín M. McManus *et al*, 2015.)

If you remember what you learned in the gut microbiome section, an unhealthy and unhappy gut is a bad thing. One of the big reasons is an unhappy gut is thought to contribute to a leaky blood brain barrier. And a leaky blood brain barrier can let bad guys into The Holy of Holies. Which again brings the whole conversation back around to nutrition as the most important part of protecting anyone's brain. A nutritionally optimized healthy brain with a fully equipped immune system could be the biggest difference between those older brains with a small infection burden and a brain of similar age, maybe even younger, that has dementia and is full of infection.

I could not find any evidence that anyone has done a clinical trial to determine if treating dementia patients with antifungals and antibiotics makes any difference.[260] (Ruth Alonso et al, 2018.) I, myself, have treated my patients who have cognitive impairment with antifungals for other problems over the years, such as thrush. Again, no one got miraculously better. I would place such therapy in the prevention category, if at all.

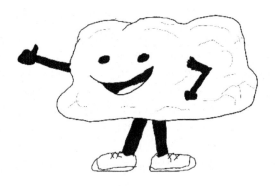

Conclusion

Dementia is truly terrifying. I have seen it both personally and professionally. Everyone knows someone who is either struggling with the disease directly or struggling with caring for a loved one who has been stricken with it. It is awful. But I say again to you with all of the hope and faith in my heart that it can be prevented. And for those of you who are struggling with the beginnings of memory loss, do not despair, do not give in, do not go gently into that grey fog from which you will never return.

I have done my best to give you a program which you can start doing today, right now, with no added testing, no added crazy fistful of pills you must take before you can get better. Just eat your veggies, exercise, chill out and get a good night's sleep. Radical stuff, I know, but it works.

There is a fifth element I have yet to address: patience. Rome was not built in a day, and neither was your disease. While the blood work for laboratory testing can take as little as seven days to show improvement with programs like ours, it can take months to start to experience real differences in memory.

One of the early adopters of our program hit the exercise portion really hard, building himself up physically to the point at which he spent a couple of hours daily on an exercise bike. He cleaned up his diet, took his sleep seriously, too. After a few months, he went on record as saying he felt great, better than he had in years. And yet his family re-ported his memory hadn't recovered. It had stopped getting worse, which was wonderful. And I had warned them it might take up to six months before the brain completely shifted into recovery mode and tried to heal. Unfortunately, he moved away and we lost track of him.

"Gosh, Cliff. What a useless story, why tell it? I'll spend hours chained to a bike and still never get better. Thanks for nothing."

I tell that story to you and my patients to illustrate that this is not a quick fix. It will take time and dedication. It will not NOT take willpower, because we all run out of willpower eventually. It will take dedication to keep making the hard choices; it will take a decision to eat the broccoli when you would rather have a bacon double cheese-burger. And make the same decision tomorrow. Next week. Next year. Five years from now.

You must choose daily to make the decisions that will unmake the lifetime of bad decisions we all make before we know better. The good news is now we know better, and it will not take another thirty years to undo the damage of the first thirty. It might take as little as three months. Maybe six months. Six months to get some hope back, to see some light through the fog. Can I promise you that all will be well and you will be completely healed? No, I cannot promise you that. But I can promise you that if you do nothing, the same six months will still slide by and you will be worse. There is no hope in doing nothing. You will only lose yourself and burden your loved ones. That I can guarantee.

I also want you to remember you don't have to get everything perfect right now. That is impossible. Do not set yourself up for failure that way. Small changes consistently implemented and followed will move mountains. Make a few changes this week. Next week make a few more. The week after that make a few more, but don't drop the changes from before. Keep building, keep finding ways to make it fun. Go with the blind faith of a communist that this collection of mustard seeds will grow and blossom in your life.

It is completely cliché to say that this is not a diet, it's a lifestyle. So, I will not say it. It is your prescription. And like all prescriptions and treatment protocols, it will only work when it is followed. If you have pneumonia, holding onto the bottle of antibiotics and memorizing the label will not get you better. Taking the pills every day and finishing the bottle is the only way it will work. It is said, faith without works is dead. This is a true saying worthy of your time and attention. This program, this prescription is more powerful than any pill out there. But it must be followed every day, or it is useless.

I know it will be hard. I know it will be difficult. I know you will make mistakes and fall off the wagon. I know I do it all the time. But what I have learned is that there is no wagon, just a path to follow toward your goals. So, if you have an imperfect day, week, month, just brush yourself off and keep going. Our enemy, dementia, will crush us if we quit. It's only by working the program and keep on keeping on do we have any chance of beating it.

If you will remember at the beginning of the book, I was losing all hope in treating my poor sick dementia patients, growing weary and even thinking of dropping out of medicine completely at times. But doing my research, cobbling together this program and actually helping people have renewed me. I now love offering hope to patients and their families.

And I am so thrilled you read the book all the way here to the end! Thank you so much. It means the world to me.

I know you have questions, and I want to answer them. Please contact us at www.keepingyourmarbles.info. We would love to hear from you.

And again, thank you. Now go out there and get to work.

Appendix A

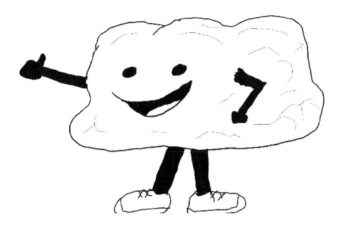

Weekly Checklist

- **Exercise**
    - ○ At least thirty minutes of aerobic exercise five days this week?
    - ○ Three sessions of strength training per week?

- **Diet**: this is a sure-fire way to get loads of nutrients and stay satisfied every day
    - ○ Smoothie or plant-based breakfast like oats
    - ○ Giant Salad for lunch including every vegetable you can handle

- A Grain, a bean and a Green for dinner like brown rice, black beans and spinach covered in Addicting Queso

(See Appendix B for further resources.)

- **Stress**
  - Meditation for ten minutes at least five out of seven days?
  - Breathing exercises at least five out of seven days?

- **Sleep**
  - No screens thirty minutes before bed every night?
  - No caffeine after noon?
  - Getting at least seven hours of sleep at night?

Appendix B
Additional Resources

Exercise
For much more on isometric exercises, I highly recommend
- *Power Isometric Isotonic Method* by Marlon Birch
- *The Charles Atlas® "Dynamic-Tension®" Bodybuilding and Fitness Course* by Charles Atlas
- *Isometrics* by Henry Wittenberg

Diet
Books

- *Seven Day Rescue Diet* by Rip Esselstyn
- *How Not To Die* By Micheal Greger
- *The Plant Based Athlete* by Matt Frazier & Robert Cheeke
- *Sick to Fit* by Josh LaJaunie (Excellent for beginners and those with 200+ pounds to lose)
- *The secrets to ultimate weight loss* by Chef AJ

Documentaries

- *Forks over Knives* to understand the health benefits and why it is a good idea to shield yourself from animal protein as best you can.
- *The Game Changers* by James Cameron and Arnold Schwarznegger. Meeting visionary scientists and top athletes, a UFC fighter embarks on a quest to find the optimal diet for human performance and health.

<u>Website</u>
- <u>nutritionfacts.org</u> is an enormous repository of videos and articles by Dr Michael Greger highlighting what the actual science says about what you should or should not eat. All explained in layman's terms with a hearty dose of humor.

Stress
<u>Books</u>
- *The Wim Hoff Method* by Wim Hoff
- *10% Happier* by Dan Harris
- *Meditation for fidgety skeptics* by Dan Harris

<u>Apps/Programs</u>
- *Headspace*, founded by Andi Puddicombe. This is the program my kids and I use everyday. It has been very helpful to me. Find it on the app store or at <u>www.headspace.com.</u>

- *Calm* is another brilliant meditation program/app with a huge amount of content designed to make you happier and less stressed. Find it on the app store or at www.calm.com.
- 10% Happier is designed for skeptical folks who are still interested in what meditation can do for them. Find it on the app store or at tenpercent.com.

Sleep
Books

- *The Sleep Revolution* by Arianna Huffington
- *Why We Sleep* by Dr Matthew Walker

Apps/Programs

All of the apps/programs in the Stress section have a great deal to say about sleep, and they all have programs to help you understand sleep a bit better and get a better night's rest.

End Notes

[1] Dale Bredesen. *The End of Alzheimer's: The First Program to Prevent and Reverse Cognitive Decline.* New York: Avery Press, 2017.

[2] Cameron J. Holloway, Lowri E. Cochlin, Yasmo Emmanuel, Andrew Murray, Ion Codreanu, Lindsay M. Edwards, Cezary Szmigielski, Damian J. Tyler, Nicholas S. Knight, Brian K. Saxby, Bridget Lambert, Campbell Thompson, Stefan Neubauer and Kieran Clarke. "A High-Fat Diet Impairs Cardiac High-Energy Phosphate Metabolism and Cognitive Function in Healthy Human Subjects." *American Journal of Clinical Nutrition,* April 2011.

[3] Lindsay M. Edwards, Andrew J. Murray, Cameron J. Holloway, Emma E. Carter, Graham J. Kemp, Ion Codreanu, Helen Brooker, Damian J. Tyler, Peter A. Robbins and Kieran Clarke. "Short-term Consumption of a High-fat Diet Impairs Whole-Body Efficiency and Cognitive Function in Sedentary Men." *Federation of American Societies for Experimental Biology Journal,* March 2011.

[4] Auriel A. Willette and Dimitrios Kapogiannis. "Does the Brain Shrink as the Waist Expands?" *Ageing Research Reviews,* 2015.

[5] Luigi Ferrucci and Elisa Fabbri. "Inflammageing: Chronic Inflammation in Ageing, Cardiovascular Disease, and Frailty." *Nature Reviews. Cardiology,* 2018.

[6] Wen-Juan Huang, Xia Zhang and Wei-Wei Chen. "Role of Oxidative Stress in Alzheimer's Disease." *Biomedical Reports,* 2016.

[7] Limor Raz, Janice Knoefel and Kiran Bhaskar. "The Neuropathology and Cerebrovascular Mechanisms of Dementia." *Journal of Cerebral Blood Flow and Metabolism,* 2016.

[8] Pedro M. Pimentel-Coelho and Serge Rivest. "The Early Contribution of Cerebrovascular Factors to the Pathogenesis of Alzheimer's Disease." *European Journal of Neuroscience*, 2012.

[9] Alios Alzheimer, Rainulf A. Stelzman, H. Norman Schnitzlein and F. Reed Murtagh. "An English Translation of Alzheimer's 1907 Paper 'Uber eine eigenartige Erkankung d Hirnrinde.'" *Clinical Anatomy*, 1995.

[10] No authors listed. "Cardiogenic Dementia." *The Lancet*, 1977.

[11] Alex E. Roher, Suzanne L. Tyas, Chera L. Maarouf, Ian D. Daugs, Tyler A. Kokjohn, Mark R. Emmerling, Zsolt Garami, Marek Belohlavek, Marwan N. Sabbagh, Lucia I. Sue and Thomas G. Beach. "Intracranial Atherosclerosis as a Contributing Factor to Alzheimer's Disease Dementia." *Alzheimer's & Dementia*, 2011.

[12] Zoe Arvanitakis, Ana W. Capuano, Sue E. Leurgans, David A. Bennett and Julie A. Schneider. "Relation of Cerebral Vessel Disease to Alzheimer's Disease, Dementia and Cognitive Function in Elderly People: A Cross-Sectional Study." *Lancet Neurology*, 2016.

[13] Jie Zhu, Yanjiang Wang, Jing Li, Juan Deng and Huadong Zhu. "Intracranial Artery Stenosis and Progression from Mild Cognitive Impairment to Alzheimer Disease." *Neurology*, 2014.

[14] Aliza P. Wingo, Wen Fan, Duc M. Duong, Ekaterina S. Gerasimov, Eric B. Dammer, Yue Liu, Nadia V. Harerimana, Bartholomew White, Madhav Thambisetty, Juan C. Troncoso, Namhee Kim, Julie A. Schneider, Ihab M. Hajjar, James J. Lah, David A. Bennett, Nicholas T. Seyfried, Allan I. Levey and Thomas S. Wingo. "Shared Proteomic Effects of Cerebral Atherosclerosis and Alzheimer's Disease on the Human Brain." *Nature Neuroscience*, 2020.

[15] Yan Deschaintre, Florence Richard, Didier Leys and Florence Pasquier. "Treatment of Vascular Risk Factors Is Associated with Slower Decline in Alzheimer Disease." *Neurology*, 2009.

[16] Geert Jan Biessels and Florin Despa. "Cognitive Decline and Dementia in Diabetes Mellitus: Mechanisms and Clinical Implications." *Nature Reviews Endocrinology*, 2018.

[17] Alison Goldin, Joshua A. Beckman, Ann Marie Schmidt and Mark A. Creager. "Advanced Glycation End Products: Sparking the Development of Diabetic Vascular Injury." *Circulation*, 2006.

[18] Haruo Hanyu. "Diabetes-Related Dementia." *Advances in Experimental Medicine and Biology*, 2019.

[19] Steven E. Arnold, Zoe Arvanitakis, Shannon L. Macauley-Rambach, Aaron M. Koenig, Hoau-Yan Wang, Rexford S. Ahima, Suzanne Craft, Sam Gandy, Christoph Buettner, Luke E. Stoeckel, David M. Holtzman and David M. Nathan. "Brain Insulin Resistance in Type 2 Diabetes and Alzheimer Disease: Concepts and Conundrums." *Nature Reviews Neurology*, 2018.

[20] Graydon S. Meneilly and Daniel M. Tessier. "Diabetes, Dementia and Hypoglycemia." *Canadian Journal of Diabetes*, 2016.

[21] Dean and Ayesha Sherzai. *The Alzheimer's Solution: A Breakthrough Program to Prevent and Reverse the Symptoms of Cognitive Decline at Every Age.* Harper One, 2017.

[22] Laia Jofre-Monseny, Anne-Marie Minihane and Gerald Rimbach. "Impact of apoE Genotype on Oxidative Stress, Inflammation and Disease Risk." *Molecular Nutrition & Food Research*, 2008.

[23] W. B. Grant. "Dietary Links to Alzheimer's Disease: 1999 Update. *Journal of Alzheimer's Disease*, 1999.

[24] Lon White, Helen Petrovitch, G. Webster Ross, Kamal H. Masaki, Robert D. Abbott, Evelyn L. Teng, Beatriz L. Rodriguez,

Patricia L. Blanchette, Richard J. Havlik, Gilbert Wergowske, Darryl Chiu, Daniel J. Foley, Carolyn Murdaugh and J. David Curb. (1996). "Prevalence of Dementia in Older Japanese-American Men in Hawaii: The Honolulu-Asia Aging Study." *JAMA: Journal of the American Medical Association, 1996.*

[25] William B. Grant. "Using Multicountry Ecological and Observational Studies to Determine Dietary Risk Factors for Alzheimer's Disease." *Journal of the American College of Nutrition,* 2016.

[26] William Montgomery, Kaname Ueda, Margaret Jorgensen, Shari Stathis, Yuanyuan Cheng and Tomomi Nakamura. "Epidemiology, Associated Burden, and Current Clinical Practice for the Diagnosis and Management of Alzheimer's Disease in Japan." *ClinicoEconomics and Outcomes Research,* 2017.

[27] Yasuhiko Saito, Jung Ki Kim, Shieva Davarian, Aaron Hagedorn and Eileen M. Crimmins. "Cognitive Performance Among Older Persons in Japan and the United States." *Journal of the American Geriatrics Society,* 2020.

[28] Michael Greger and Gene Stone. *How Not to Die.* Flatiron Books, 2015.

[29] B. Sepehrnia, M. I. Kamboh, L. L. Adams-Campbell, C. H. Bunker, M. Nwankwo, P. P. Majumder and R. E. Ferrell. "Genetic Studies of Human Apolipoproteins. X. The Effect of the Apolipoprotein E Polymorphism on Quantitative Levels of Lipoproteins in Nigerian Blacks." *American Journal of Human Genetics,* 1989.

[30] William B. Grant. "Dietary Links to Alzheimer's Disease: 1999 Update." *Journal of Alzheimer's Disease,* 1999.

[31] Miia Kivipelto, Eeva-Liisa Helkala, Mikko P. Laakso, Tuomo Hänninen, Merja Hallikainen, Kari Alhainen, Susan Livonen, Arto Mannermaa, Jaakko Tuomilehto, Aulikki Nissinen and Hikka Soininen. "Apolipoprotein E Epsilon4 Allele, Elevated Midlife

Total Cholestrol Level, and High Midlife Systolic Blood Pressure Are Independent Risk Factors for Late-Life Alzheimer's Disease." *Annals of Internal Medicine,* 2002.

[32] American Geriatrics Society Beers Criteria® Update Expert Panel. Updated AGS Beers Criteria® for Potentially Inappropriate Medication Use in Older Adults. *Journal of the American Geriatrics Society,* 2019.

[33] Carol A. C. Coupland, Trevor Hill, Tom Dening, Richard Morriss, Michael Moore and Julia Hippisley-Cox. "Anticholinergic Drug Exposure and the Risk of Dementia." *JAMA Internal Medicine,* 2019.

[34] Bjørn Erik Neerland, Maria Krogseth, Vibeke Juliebø, Anette Hylen Ranhoff, Knut Engedal, Frede Frihagen, Johan Ræder, Torgeir Bruun Wyller and Leiv Otto Watne. "Perioperative Hemodynamics and Risk for Delirium and New Onset Dementia in Hip Fracture Patients; A Prospective Follow-up Study." *PLoS One,* 2017.

[35] Terry E. Goldberg, Chen Chen, Yuanjia Wang, Eunice Jung, Antoinette Swanson, Caleb Ing, Paul S. Garcia, Robert A. Whittington and Vivek Moitra. "Association of Delirium with Long-term Cognitive Decline: A Meta-analysis." *JAMA Neurology,* 2020.

[36] C. Courtney, D. Farrell, R. Gray, R. Hills, L. Lynch, E. Sellwood, S. Edwards, W. Hardyman, J. Raftery, P. Crome, C. Lendon, H. Shaw, P. Bentham and AD2000 Collaborative Group. "Long-Term Donepezil Treatment in 565 Patients with Alzheimer's Disease (AD2000): Randomised Double-Blind Trial." *The Lancet,* 2004.

[37] Jacqueline S. Birks and Richard J. Harvey. "Donepezil for Dementia Due to Alzheimer's Disease." *Cochrane Database Systematic Reviews,* 2018.

[38] David S. Knopman and Joel S. Perlmutter. "Prescribing Aducanumab in the Face of Meager Efficacy and Real Risks." *Neurology*, 2021.

[39] Michael F. Egan, James Kost, Tiffini Voss, Yuki Mukai, Paul S. Aisen, Jeffrey L. Cummings, Pierre N. Tariot, Bruno Vellas, Christopher H. van Dyck, Merce Boada, Ying Zhang, Wen Li, Christine Furtek, Erin Mahoney, Lyn Harper Mozley, Yi Mo, Cyrille Sur and David Michelson. "Randomized Trial of Verubecestat for Prodromal Alzheimer's Disease." *The New England Journal of Medicine*, 2019.

[40] https://www.wsj.com/articles/biogen-cuts-price-for-alzheimers-drug-aduhelm-byhalf-11640001661

[41] https://www.bbc.com/news/health-59699907

[42] https://www.statnews.com/2022/01/11/medicare-aduhelm-proposeddecision/

[43] Elisabeth Mahase. "Aducanumab: European Agency Rejects Alzheimer's Drug Over Efficacy and Safety Concerns." *The BMJ*, 2021.

[44] P. Giem, W. L. Beeson and G. E. Fraser. "The Incidence of Dementia and Intake of Animal Products: Preliminary Findings from the Adventist Health Study." *Neuroepidemiology*, 1993.

[45] Wei Xu, Lan Tan, Hui-Fu Wang, Teng Jiang, Meng-Shan Tan, Lin Tan, Qing-Fei Zhao, Jie-Qiong Li, Jun Wang and Jin-Tai Yu. "Meta-Analysis of Modifiable Risk Factors for Alzheimer's Disease." *Journal of Neurology, Neurosurgery & Psychiatry*, 2015.

[46] Lap Tai Le and Joan Sabaté. "Beyond Meatless, the Health Effects of Vegan Diets: Findings from the Adventist Cohorts." *Nutrients*, 2014.

[47] https://www.hsph.harvard.edu/nutritionsource/

[48] Tiia Ngandu, Jenni Lehtisalo, Alina Solomon, Esko Levälahti, Satu Ahtiluoto, Riitta Antikainen, Lars Bäckman, Tuomo Hänninen, Antti Jula, Tiina Laatikainen, Jaana Lindström, Francesca Mangialasche, Teemu Paajanen, Satu Pajala, Markku Peltonen, Rainer Rauramaa, Anna Stigsdotter-Neely, Timo Strandberg, Jaakko Tuomilehto, Hilkka Soininen and Miia Kivipelto. "A 2 Year Multidomain Intervention of Diet, Exercise, Cognitive Training, and Vascular Risk Monitoring Versus Control to Prevent Cognitive Decline in At-Risk Elderly People (FINGER): a Randomised Controlled Trial." *The Lancet*, 2015.

[49] Anna Rosenberg, Tiia Ngandu, Minna Rusanen, Riitta Antikainen, Lars Bäckman, Satu Havulinna, Tuomo Hänninen, Tiina Laatikainen, Jenni Lehtisalo, Esko Levälahti, Jaana Lindström, Teemu Paajanen, Markku Peltonen, Hilkka Soininen, Anna Stigsdotter-Neely, Timo Strandberg, Jaakko Tuomilehto, Alina Solomon and Miia Kivipelto. "Multidomain Lifestyle Intervention Benefits a Large Elderly Population at Risk for Cognitive Decline and Dementia Regardless of Baseline Characteristics: The FINGER Trial." *Alzheimer's & Dementia*, 2018.

[50] Hai-Qiang Li, Long Tan, Hong-Peng Yang, Wei Pang, Tong Xu and Yu-Gang Jiang. "Changes of Hippocampus Proteomic Profiles After Blueberry Extracts Supplementation in APP/PS1 Transgenic Mice." *Nutritional Neuroscience*, 2020

[51] Erin L. Boespflug, James C. Eliassen, Jonathan A. Dudley, Marcelle D. Shidler, Wilhelmina Kalt, Suzanne S. Summer, Amanda L. Stein, Amanda N. Stover and Robert Krikorian. "Enhanced Neural Activation with Blueberry Supplementation in Mild Cognitive Impairment." *Nutritional Neuroscience*, 2018.

[52] Felice N. Jacka, Nicolas Cherbuin, Kaarin J. Anstey, Perminder Sachdev and Peter Butterworth. "Western Diet is Associated with a Smaller Hippocampus: A Longitudinal Investigation." *BMC Medicine*, 2015.

[53] Tuki Attuquayefio, Richard J. Stevenson, Megan J. Oaten and Heather M. Francis. "A Four-Day Western-Style Dietary Intervention Causes Reductions in Hippocampal-Dependent Learning and Memory and Interoceptive Sensitivity." *PLoS One*, 2017.

[54] Yu-Chen Cheng, Jer-Ming Sheen, Wen Long Hu and Yu-Chiang Hung. "Polyphenols and Oxidative Stress in Atherosclerosis-Related Ischemic Heart Disease and Stroke." *Oxidative Medicine and Cellular Longevity*, 2017.

[55] Susanne Rautiainen, Susanna Larsson, Jarmo Virtamo and Alicja Wolk. "Total Antioxidant Capacity of Diet and Risk of Stroke: A Population-Based Prospective Cohort of Women." *Stroke*, 2012.

[56] Alex E. Roher, Suzanne L. Tyas, Chera L. Maarouf, Ian D. Daugs, Tyler A. Kokjohn, Mark R. Emmerling, Zsolt Garami, Marek Belohlavek, Marwan N. Sabbagh, Lucia I. Sue and Thomas G. Beach. "Intracranial Atherosclerosis as a Contributing Factor to Alzheimer's Disease Dementia." *Alzheimer's & Dementia*, 2011.

[57] Dean Ornish, S. E. Brown, Larry W. Scherwitz, James H. Billings, William T. Armstrong, Thomas A. Ports, S. M. McLanahan, Richard L. Kirkeeide, Richard J. Brand and K. Lance Gould. "Can Lifestyle Changes Reverse Coronary Heart Disease? The Lifestyle Heart Trial." *The Lancet*, 1990.

[58] Caldwell B. Esselstyn, Jr., Gina Gendy, Jonathan Doyle, Mladen Golubic and Michael F. Roizen. "A Way to Reverse CAD?" *The Journal of Family Practice*, 2014.

[59] Dean Ornish, Larry W. Scherwitz, James H. Billings, S. E. Brown, K. Lance Gould, Terri A. Merritt, Stephen Sparler, William T. Armstrong, Thomas A. Ports, Richard L. Kirkeeide, Charissa Hogeboom and Richard J. Brand. "Intensive Lifestyle Changes for Reversal of Coronary Heart Disease." *JAMA*, 1998.

[60] Hsin-Chia Hung, Kaumudi J. Joshipura, Rui Jiang, Frank B. Hu, David Hunter, Stephanie A. Smith-Warner, Graham A. Colditz, Bernard Rosner, Donna Spiegelman and Walter C. Willett. "Fruit and Vegetable Intake and Risk of Major Chronic Disease." *Journal of the National Cancer Institute*, 2004.

[61] Phillip Tuso, Scott R. Stoll and William W. Li. "A Plant-Based Diet, Atherogenesis, and Coronary Artery Disease Prevention." *The Permanente Journal*, 2015.

[62] Alicja Wolk. "Potential Health Hazards of Eating Red Meat." *Journal of Internal Medicine*, 2017.

[63] Caldwell B. Esselstyn, Jr. "Updating a 12-Year Experience with Arrest and Reversal Therapy for Coronary Heart Disease (An Overdue Requiem for Palliative Cardiology)." *The American Journal of Cardiology*, 1999.

[64] Michael Greger. "A Whole Food Plant-Based Diet is Effective for Weight Loss: The Evidence." *American Journal of Lifestyle Medicine*, 2020

[65] Binita Shah, Jonathan D. Newman, Kathleen Woolf, Lisa Ganguzza, Yu Guo, Nicole Allen, Judy Zhong, Edward A. Fisher and James Slater. "Anti-Inflammatory Effects of a Vegan Diet Versus the American Heart Association-Recommended Diet in Coronary Artery Disease Trial." *Journal of the American Heart Association*, 2018.

[66] Olivia I. Okereke, Bernard A. Rosner, Dae H. Kim, Jae H. Kang, Nancy R. Cook, JoAnn E. Manson, Julie E. Buring, Walter C. Willett and Francine Grodstein. "Dietary Fat Types and 4-Year Cognitive Change in Community-Dwelling Older Women." *Annals of Neurology*, 2012.

[67] Salvatore Mottillo, Kristian B. Filion, Jacques Genest, Lawrence Joseph, Louise Pilote, Paul Poirier, Stéphane Rinfret, Ernesto L. Schiffrin and Mark J. Eisenberg. "The Metabolic Syndrome and Cardiovascular Risk a Systematic Review and Meta-Analysis." *Journal of the American College of Cardiology*, 2010.

[68] John T. Brosnan. "Comments on Metabolic Needs for Glucose and the Role of Gluconeogenesis." *European Journal of Clinical Nutrition*, 1999.

[69] Susanne H. Holt, Janette C. Miller and Peter Petocz. "An Insulin Index of Foods: The Insulin Demand Generated by 1000-kJ Portions of Common Foods." *The American Journal of Clinical Nutrition*, 1997.

[70] J. Denis McGarry. "Banting Lecture 2001: Dysregulation of Fatty Acid Metabolism in the Etiology of Type 2 Diabetes." *Diabetes*, 2002.

[71] Michael Roden, Thomas B. Price, Gianluca Perseghin, Kitt Falk Petersen, Douglas L. Rothman, Gary W. Cline and Gerald I. Shulman. "Mechanism of Free Fatty Acid-Induced Insulin Resistance in Humans." *The Journal of Clinical Investigation*, 1996.

[72] Michael Roden, Martin Krssak, Harald Stingl, Stephan Gruber, A. Hofer, Clemens Fürnsinn, Ewald Moser and Werner Klaus Waldhäusl. "Rapid Impairment of Skeletal Muscle Glucose Transport/Phosphorylation by Free Fatty Acids in Humans." *Diabetes*, 1999.

[73] Dawn K. Coletta and Lawrence J. Mandarino. "Mitochondrial Dysfunction and Insulin Resistance from the Outside in: Extracellular Matrix, the Cytoskeleton, and Mitochondria." *American Journal of Physiology: Endocrinology and Metabolism*, 2011.

[74] Christopher J. Nolan and Claire Z. Larter. "Lipotoxicity: Why do Saturated Fatty Acids Cause and Monounsaturates Protect Against It?" *Journal of Gastroenterology and Hepatology*, 2009.

[75] Gianluca Perseghin, Paola Scifo, Francesco De Cobelli, Emanuela Pagliato, Alberto Battezzati, Cinzia Arcelloni, Angelo Vanzulli, Giulio Testolin, Guido Pozza, Alessandro Del Maschio and Livio Luzi. "Intramyocellular Triglyceride Content is a Determinant of in Vivo Insulin Resistance in Humans: a 1H-13C Nuclear Magnetic Resonance Spectroscopy Assessment in Offspring of Type 2 Diabetic Parents." *Diabetes*, 1999.

[76] Christopher J. Nolan and Claire Z. Larter. "Lipotoxicity: Why do Saturated Fatty Acids Cause and Monounsaturates Protect Against It?" *Journal of Gastroenterology and Hepatology*, 2009.

[77] Suzanne M. de la Monte. "Type 3 Diabetes is Sporadic Alzheimer's Disease: Mini-Review." *European Neuropsychopharmacology*, 2014

[78] Adina C. Bosch, Bernadette O'Neill, Gunnar O. Sigge, Sven E. Kerwath and Louwrens C. Hoffman. "Heavy Metals in Marine Fish Meat and Consumer Health: A Review." *Journal of the Science of Food and Agriculture*, 2016.

[79] Jin-Ling Liu, Xiang-Rong Xu, Zhen-Hua Ding, Jia-Xi Peng, Ming-Hua Jin, You-Shao Wang, Yi-Guo Hong and Wei-Zhong Yue. "Heavy Metals in Wild Marine Fish from South China Sea: Levels, Tissue- and Species-Specific Accumulation and Potential Risk to Humans." *Ecotoxicology*, 2015.

[80] Akshay Goel, Naga Venkata Pothineni, Mayank Singhal, Hakan Paydak, Tom Saldeen and Jawahar L. Mehta. "Fish, Fish Oils and Cardioprotection: Promise or Fish Tale?" *International Journal of Molecular Sciences*, 2018.

[81] Gina Segovia-Siapco and Joan Sabaté. "Health and Sustainability Outcomes of Vegetarian Dietary Patterns: A Revisit of the EPIC-Oxford and the Adventist Health Study-2 Cohorts." *European Journal of Clinical Nutrition*, 2019.

[82] Faidon Magkos, Fotini Arvaniti and Antonis Zampelas. "Organic Food: Nutritious Food or Food for Thought? A Review of the Evidence." *International Journal of Food Sciences and Nutrition*, 2003.

[83] Faidon Magkos, Fotini Arvaniti and Antonis Zampelas. "Organic Food: Buying More Safety or Just Peace of Mind? A Critical Review of the Literature." *Critical Reviews in Food Science and Nutrition*, 2006.

[84] Anna Lindén, Kristina Andersson and Agneta Oskarsson. "Cadmium in Organic and Conventional Pig Production." *Archives of Environmental Contamination and Toxicology*, 2001.

[85] K. E. Bradbury, A. Balkwill, E. A. Spencer, A. W. Roddam, G. K. Reeves, J. Green, T. J. Key, V. Beral, K. Pirie and The Million Women Study Collaborators. "Organic Food Consumption and the Incidence of Cancer in a Large Prospective Study of Women in the United Kingdom." *British Journal of Cancer*, 2014.

[86] Fabrizio Giannandrea, Loredana Gandini, Donatella Paoli, Roberta Turci and Irene Figà-Talamanca. "Pesticide Exposure and Serum Organochlorine Residuals Among Testicular Cancer Patients and Healthy Controls." *Journal of Environmental Science and Health Part B*, 2011.

[87] Ria Chhabra, Santharam Kolli and Johannes H. Bauer. "Organically Grown Food Provides Health Benefits to Drosophila Melanogaster." *PLoS One*, 2013.

[88] Richard Reiss, Jason Johnston, Kevin Tucker, John M. DeSesso and Carl L. Keen. "Estimation of Cancer Risks and Benefits Associated with a Potential Increased Consumption of Fruits and Vegetables." *Food and Chemical Toxicology*, 2012.

[89] U.S. Department of Health and Human Services. *Physical Activity Guidelines for Americans, 2nd edition*. Washington, DC: U.S. Department of Health and Human Services, 2018.

[90] Laura D. Baker, Laura L. Frank, Karen Foster-Schubert, Pattie S. Green, Charles W. Wilkinson, Anne McTiernan, Stephen R. Plymate, Mark A. Fishel, G. Stennis Watson, Brenna A. Cholerton, Glen E. Duncan, Pankaj D. Mehta and Suzanne Craft. "Effects of Aerobic Exercise on Mild Cognitive Impairment: A Controlled Trial." *Archives of Neurology*, 2010.

[91] Kirk I. Erickson, Michelle W. Voss, Ruchika Shaurya Prakash, Chandramallika Basak, Amanda Szabo, Laura Chaddock, Jennifer S. Kim, Susie Heo, Heloisa Alves, Siobhan M. White, Thomas R. Wojcicki, Emily Mailey, Victoria J. Vieira, Stephen A. Martin, Brandt D. Pence, Jeffrey A. Woods, Edward McAuley and Arthur F. Kramer. "Exercise Training Increases Size of Hippocampus and Improves Memory." *Proceedings of the National Academy of Sciences*, 2011.

[92] Nicole C. L. Hess and Neil A. Smart. "Isometric Exercise Training for Managing Vascular Risk Factors in Mild Cognitive Impairment and Alzheimer's Disease." *Frontiers in Aging Neuroscience*, 2017.

[93] Paul G. Peters, Helaine M. Alessio, Ann E. Hagerman, Tony Ashton, Szilvia Nagy and Ronald L. Wiley. "Short-Term Isometric Exercise Reduces Systolic Blood Pressure in Hypertensive Adults: Possible Role of Reactive Oxygen Species." *International Journal of Cardiology*, 2006.

[94] Broino Kiveloff and Olive Huber. "Brief Maximal Isometric Exercise in Hypertension." *Journal of the American Geriatrics Society*, 1971.

[95] David E. Fixler, W. Pennock Laird, Richard Browne, Victoria Fitzgerald, Susan Wilson and Ruth Vance. "Response of Hypertensive Adolescents to Dynamic and Isometric Exercise Stress." *Pediatrics*, 1979.

[96] Ashley Carvalho, Irene Maeve Rea, Tanyalak Parimon and Barry J. Cusack. "Physical Activity and Cognitive Function in Individuals

Over 60 Years of Age: A Systematic Review." *Clinical Interventions in Aging*, 2014.

[97] Sarah E. Lamb, Dipesh Mistry, Sharisse Alleyne, Nicky Atherton, Deborah Brown, Bethan Copsey, Sukhdeep Dosanjh, Susanne Finnegan, Beth Fordham, Frances Griffiths, Susie Hennings, Iftekhar Khan, Kamran Khan, Ranjit Lall, Samantha Lyle, Vivien Nichols, Stavros Petrou, Peter Zeh and Bart Sheehan. "Aerobic and Strength Training Exercise Programme for Cognitive Impairment in People with Mild to Moderate Dementia: The DAPA RCT." *Health Technology Assessment*, 2018.

[98] Th. Hettinger and E. Müller. "Muskelleistung und Muskeltraining [Muscle Capacity and Muscle Training]." *Arbeitsphysiologie*, 1953.

[99] Sophia Bennett and Alan J. Thomas. "Depression and Dementia: Cause, Consequence or Coincidence?" *Maturitas*, 2014.

[100] Breno S. Diniz, Meryl A. Butters, Steven M. Albert, Mary Amanda Dew and Charles F. Reynolds 3rd. "Late-Life Depression and Risk of Vascular Dementia and Alzheimer's Disease: Systematic Review and Meta-Analysis of Community-Based Cohort Studies." *The British Journal of Psychiatry*, 2013.

[101] Arash Salardini. "An Overview of Primary Dementias as Clinicopathological Entities." *Seminars in Neurology*, 2019.

[102] Thomas W. Meeks, Susan A. Ropacki and Dilip V. Jeste. "The Neurobiology of Neuropsychiatric Syndromes in Dementia." *Current Opinion in Psychiatry*, 2006.

[103] H. Gutzmann and A. Qazi. "Depression Associated with Dementia." *Zeitschrift für Gerontologie und Geriatrie*, 2015.

[104] Peter J. Carek, Sarah E. Laibstain and Stephen M. Carek. "Exercise for the Treatment of Depression and Anxiety." *International Journal of Psychiatry in Medicine*, 2011.

[105] Andreas Ströhle. "Physical Activity, Exercise, Depression and Anxiety Disorders." *Journal of Neural Transmission (Vienna)*, 2009.

[106] Bonnie L. Beezhold, Carol S. Johnston and Deanna R. Daigle. "Vegetarian Diets are Associated with Healthy Mood States: A Cross-Sectional Study in Seventh Day Adventist Adults." *Nutrition Journal*, 2010.

[107] Bonnie L. Beezhold and Carol S. Johnston. "Restriction of Meat, Fish, and Poultry in Omnivores Improves Mood: A Pilot Randomized Controlled Trial." *Nutrition Journal*, 2012.

[108] Yousef Sawikr, Nagendra Sastry Yarla, Ilaria Peluso, Mohammad Amjad Kamal, Gjumrakch Aliev and Anupam Bishayee. "Neuroinflammation in Alzheimer's Disease: The Preventive and Therapeutic Potential of Polyphenolic Nutraceuticals." *Advances in Protein Chemistry Structural Biology*, 2017.

[109] Fernando Gomez-Pinilla and Trang T. J. Nguyen. "Natural Mood Foods: The Actions of Polyphenols Against Psychiatric and Cognitive Disorders." *Nutritional Neuroscience*, 2012.

[110] Tjalling Jan Holwerda, Dorly J. H. Deeg, Aartjan T. F. Beekman, Theo G. van Tilburg, Max L. Stek, Cees Jonker and Robert A. Schoevers. "Feelings of Loneliness, but not Social Isolation, Predict Dementia Onset: Results from the Amsterdam Study of the Elderly (AMSTEL)." *Journal of Neurology, Neurosurgery & Psychiatry*, 2014.

[111] Ross Penninkilampi, Anne-Nicole Casey, Maria Fiatarone Singh and Henry Brodaty. "The Association Between Social Engagement, Loneliness, and Risk of Dementia: A Systematic Review and Meta-Analysis." *Journal of Alzheimer's Disease*, 2018.

[112] M. Sol Ibarra-Rovillard and Nicholas A. Kuiper. "Social Support and Social Negativity Findings in Depression: Perceived Responsiveness to Basic Psychological Needs." *Clinical Psychology Review*, 2011.

[113] Tim D. Windsor, Denis Gerstorf, Elissa Pearson, Lindsay H. Ryan and Kaarin J. Anstey. "Positive and Negative Social Exchanges and Cognitive Aging in Young-Old Adults: Differential Associations Across Family, Friend, and Spouse Domains." *Psychology and Aging*, 2014.

[114] Raquel Vilanova Araujo, Ana Fátima Carvalho Fernandes, Inez Sampaio Nery, Elaine Maria Leite Rangel Andrade, Lídya Tolstenko Nogueira and Francisco Honeidy Carvalho Azevedo. "Meditation Effect on Psychological Stress Level in Women with Breast Cancer: A Systematic Review. Efeito da Meditação no Nível de Estresse Psicológico de Mulheres com Neoplasia Mamária: Revisão Sistemática." *Revista da Escola de Enfermagem da USP*, 2019.

[115] Rinske A. Gotink, Rozanna Meijboom, Meike W. Vernooij, Marion Smits and M. G. Myriam Hunink. "8-Week Mindfulness Based Stress Reduction Induces Brain Changes Similar to Traditional Long-Term Meditation Practice - A Systematic Review." *Brain and Cognition*, 2016.

[116] Madhuri R. Tolahunase, Rajesh Sagar, Muneeb Faiq and Rima Dada. "Yoga- and Meditation-Based Lifestyle Intervention Increases Neuroplasticity and Reduces Severity of Major Depressive Disorder: A Randomized Controlled Trial." *Restorative Neurology and Neuroscience*, 2018.

[117] Elizabeth F. Ball, Emira Nur Shafina Muhammad Sharizan, Genny Franklin and Ewelina Rogozińska. "Does Mindfulness Meditation Improve Chronic Pain? A Systematic Review." *Current Opinion in Obstetrics and Gynecology*, 2017.

[118] Jesse Russell-Williams, Wafa Jaroudi, Tania Perich, Siobhan Hoscheidt, Mohamad El Haj and Ahmed A. Moustafa. "Mindfulness and Meditation: Treating Cognitive Impairment and Reducing Stress in Dementia." *Reviews in the Neurosciences*, 2018.

[119] Wee Ping Wong, Jan Coles, Richard Chambers, David Bin-Chia Wu and Craig Hassed. "The Effects of Mindfulness on Older

Adults with Mild Cognitive Impairment." *Journal of Alzheimer's Disease Reports*, 2017.

[120] Jon Kabat-Zinn. *Wherever You Go, There You Are: Mindfulness Meditation in Everyday Life.* Hachette Books, 1994.

[121] Hui-Xia Zhou, Xiao Chen, Yang-Qian Shen, Le Li, Ning-Xuan Chen, Zhi-Chen Zhu, Francisco Xavier Castellanos and Chao-Gan Yan. "Rumination and the Default Mode Network: Meta-Analysis of Brain Imaging Studies and Implications for Depression." *NeuroImage*, 2020.

[122] Elaine Yang, Elizabeth Schamber, Rika M. L. Meyer and Jeffrey I. Gold. "Happier Healers: Randomized Controlled Trial of Mobile Mindfulness for Stress Management." *Journal of Alternative and Complementary Medicine*, 2018.

[123] Jennifer Huberty, Jeni Green, Christine Glissmann, Linda Larkey, Megan Puzia and Chong Lee. "Efficacy of the Mindfulness Meditation Mobile App "Calm" to Reduce Stress Among College Students: Randomized Controlled Trial." *JMIR mHealth and uHealth*, 2019.

[124] Richard P. Brown and Patricia L. Gerbarg. "Yoga Breathing, Meditation, and Longevity." *Annals of the New York Academy of Sciences*, 2009.

[125] Holger Cramer, Romy Lauche, Jost Langhorst and Gustav Dobos. "Yoga for Depression: A Systematic Review and Meta-Analysis." *Depression and Anxiety*, 2013.

[126] Edgar Toschi-Dias, Eleonora Tobaldini, Monica Solbiati, Giorgio Costantino, Roberto Sanlorenzo, Stefania Doria, Floriana Irtelli, Claudio Mencacci and Nicola Montano. "Sudarshan Kriya Yoga Improves Cardiac Autonomic Control in Patients with Anxiety-Depression Disorders." *Journal of Affective Disorders*, 2017.

[127] Richard P. Brown and Patricia L. Gerbarg. "Sudarshan Kriya Yogic Breathing in the Treatment of Stress, Anxiety, and Depression: Part I-Neurophysiologic Model." *Journal of Alternative and Complementary Medicine*, 2005.

[128] Lisa A. Uebelacker, Geoffrey Tremont, Lee T. Gillette, Gary Epstein-Lubow, David R. Strong, Ana M. Abrantes, Audrey R. Tyrka, Tanya Tran, Brandon A. Gaudiano and Ivan W. Miller. "Adjunctive Yoga v. Health Education for Persistent Major Depression: A Randomized Controlled Trial." *Psychological Medicine*, 2017.

[129] Alina Prax. "How to Release Anxiety Using Breath." *Yogapedia.com*, 2020.

[130] Wim Hof. *The Wim Hof Method: Activate Your Full Human Potential.* Sounds True, 2020.

[131] American Psychological Association. "What is Cognitive Behavioral Therapy?" *PTSD Guideline*, 2017.

[132] Antonia N. Kaczkurkin and Edna B. Foa. "Cognitive-Behavioral Therapy for Anxiety Disorders: An Update on the Empirical Evidence." *Dialogues in Clinical Neuroscience*, 2015.

[133] Gavin Andrews, Jill M. Newby and Alishia D. Williams. "Internet-Delivered Cognitive Behavior Therapy for Anxiety Disorders is Here to Stay." *Current Psychiatry Reports*, 2015.

[134] Sogol Javaheri, Ying Y. Zhao, Naresh M. Punjabi, Stuart F. Quan, Daniel J. Gottlieb and Susan Redline. "Slow-Wave Sleep Is Associated with Incident Hypertension: The Sleep Heart Health Study." *Sleep*, 2018.

[135] Robbert Havekes, Alan J. Park, Jennifer C. Tudor, Vincent G. Luczak, Rolf T. Hansen, Sarah L. Ferri, Vibeke M. Bruinenberg, Shane G. Poplawski, Jonathan P. Day, Sara J. Aton, Kasia Radwańska, Peter Meerlo, Miles D. Houslay, George S. Baillie and

Ted Abel. "Sleep Deprivation Causes Memory Deficits by Negatively Impacting Neuronal Connectivity in Hippocampal Area CA1." *eLife*, 2016.

[136] Jae-Eun Kang, Miranda M. Lim, Randall J. Bateman, James J. Lee, Liam P. Smyth, John R. Cirrito, Nobuhiro Fujiki, Seiji Nishino and David M. Holtzman. "Amyloid-Beta Dynamics are Regulated by Orexin and the Sleep-Wake Cycle." *Science*, 2009.

[137] Marie E. Gaine, Snehajyoti Chatterjee and Ted Abel. "Sleep Deprivation and the Epigenome." *Frontiers in Neural Circuits*, 2018.

[138] Le Shi, Si-Jing Chen, Meng-Ying Ma, Yan-Ping Bao, Ying Han, Yu-Mei Wang, Jie Shi, Michael V. Vitiello and Lin Lu. "Sleep Disturbances Increase the Risk of Dementia: A Systematic Review and Meta-Analysis." *Sleep Medicine Reviews*, 2018.

[139] Philip G. Haydon. "Astrocytes and the Modulation of Sleep." *Current Opinion in Neurobiology*, 2017.

[140] Scott Bragg, J. J. Benich, Natalie Christian, Josh Visserman and John Freedy. "Updates in Insomnia Diagnosis and Treatment." *International Journal of Psychiatry in Medicine*, 2019.

[141] 2019 American Geriatrics Society Beers Criteria® Update Expert Panel. "American Geriatrics Society 2019 Updated AGS Beers Criteria® for Potentially Inappropriate Medication Use in Older Adults." *Journal of the American Geriatrics Society*, 2019.

[142] Anne M. Holbrook, Renée Crowther, Ann Lotter, Chiachen Cheng and Derek King. "Meta-analysis of Benzodiazepine Use in the Treatment of Insomnia." *Canadian Medical Association Journal*, 2000.

[143] No authors listed. "Sleep Complaints: Whenever Possible, Avoid the Use of Sleeping Pills." *Prescrire International*, 2008.

[144] Cheryl M. Paradis, Lawrence A. Siegel and Stuart B. Kleinman. "Two Cases of Zolpidem-Associated Homicide." *The Primary Care Companion for CNS Disorders*, 2012.

[145] Paul Sadler, Suzanne McLaren, Britt Klein, Jack Harvey and Megan Jenkins. "Cognitive Behavior Therapy for Older Adults with Insomnia and Depression: A Randomized Controlled Trial in Community Mental Health Services." *Sleep*, 2018.

[146] Sadler, McLaren, Klein, Harvey and Jenkins. "Cognitive Behavior Therapy for Older Adults with Insomnia and Depression: A Randomized Controlled Trial in Community Mental Health Services."

[147] Glenna S. Brewster, Barbara Riegel and Philip R. Gehrman. "Insomnia in the Older Adult." *Sleep Medicine Clinics*, 2018.

[148 A] Centers for Disease Control and Prevention. "Tips for Better Sleep." *CDC*, 2016.

[148 B] American Academy of Sleep Medicine. "Healthy Sleep Habits." *AASM*, 2020.

[149] Shawn Bishop. "Misleading Aspirin Email." *Mayo Clinic*, 2010.

[150] Kikuo Okamura, Yukihiko Washimi, Hidetoshi Endo, Haruhiko Tokuda, Yukio Shiga, Hisayuki Miura and Yoshikatsu Nojiri. ["Can high fluid intake prevent cerebral and myocardial infarction?" Systematic review]. *Nihon Ronen Igakkai Zasshi*, 2005.

[151] Anna E. Kirkland, Gabrielle L. Sarlo and Kathleen F. Holton. "The Role of Magnesium in Neurological Disorders." *Nutrients*, 2018.

[152] Kenneth Lo, Qing Liu, Tracy Madsen, Steve Rapp, Jiu-Chiuan Chen, Marian Neuhouser, Aladdin Shadyab, Lubna Pal, Xiaochen Lin, Sally Shumaker, JoAnn Manson, Ying-Qing Feng and Simin Liu. "Relations of Magnesium Intake to Cognitive Impairment and

Dementia Among Participants in the Women's Health Initiative Memory Study: A Prospective Cohort Study." *BMJ Open*, 2019.

[153] Wen-Wen Cheng, Qiang Zhu and Hong-Yu Zhang. "Mineral Nutrition and the Risk of Chronic Diseases: A Mendelian Randomization Study." *Nutrients*, 2019.

[154] Senthilkumar Sankararaman and Thomas J. Sferra. "Are We Going Nuts on Coconut Oil?" *Current Nutrition Reports*, 2018.

[155] Taylor C. Wallace. "Health Effects of Coconut Oil-A Narrative Review of Current Evidence." *Journal of the American College of Nutrition*, 2019.

[156] Laurence Eyres, Michael F. Eyres, Alexandra Chisholm and Rachel C. Brown. "Coconut Oil Consumption and Cardiovascular Risk Factors in Humans." *Nutrition Reviews*, 2016.

[157] Alok Sharma, Marc Bemis and Alicia R. Desilets. "Role of Medium Chain Triglycerides (Axona®) in the Treatment of Mild to Moderate Alzheimer's Disease." *American Journal of Alzheimer's Disease and Other Dementias*, 2014.

[158] Mark A. Reger, Samuel T. Henderson, Cathy Hale, Brenna Cholerton, Laura D. Baker, G. S. Watson, Karen Hyde, Darla Chapman and Suzanne Craft. "Effects of Beta-Hydroxybutyrate on Cognition in Memory-Impaired Adults." *Neurobiology of Aging*, 2004.

[159] Miho Ota, Junko Matsuo, Ikki Ishida, Harumasa Takano, Yuma Yokoi, Hiroaki Hori, Sumiko Yoshida, Kinya Ashida, Kentaro Nakamura, Takeshi Takahashi and Hiroshi Kunugi. "Effects of a Medium-ChainTtriglyceride-Based Ketogenic Formula on Cognitive Function in Patients with Mild-to-Moderate Alzheimer's Disease." *Neuroscience Letters*, 2019.

[160] Qing Xu, Yong Zhang, Xinsheng Zhang, Lu Liu, Bo Zhou, Rui Mo, Yan Li, Huizi Li, Feng Li, Yang Tao, Yinghua Liu and Changyong Xue. "Medium-Chain Triglycerides Improved

Cognition and Lipid Metabolomics in Mild to Moderate Alzheimer's Disease Patients with APOE4-/-: A Double-Blind, Randomized, Placebo-Controlled Crossover Trial." *Clinical Nutrition*, 2020.

[161] Emma Sydenham, Alan D. Dangour, Wee-Shiong Lim. "Omega 3 Fatty Acid for the Prevention of Cognitive Decline and Dementia." *The Cochrane Database of Systematic Reviews*, 2012.

[162] Marion Burckhardt, Max Herke, Tobias Wustmann, Stefan Watzke, Gero Langer and Astrid Fink. "Omega-3 Fatty Acids for the Treatment of Dementia." *The Cochrane Database of Systematic Reviews*, 2016.

[163] Scheine Canhada, Kamila Castro, Ingrid Schweigert Perry and Vivian Cristine Luft. "Omega-3 Fatty Acids' Supplementation in Alzheimer's Disease: A Systematic Review." *Nutritional Neuroscience*, 2018.

[164] Noemí Esteras, Albena T. Dinkova-Kostova and Andrey Y. Abramov. "Nrf2 Activation in the Treatment of Neurodegenerative Diseases: A Focus on its Role in Mitochondrial Bioenergetics and Function." *Biological Chemistry*, 2016.

[165] Kelsey E. Murphy and Joshua J. Park. "Can Co-Activation of Nrf2 and Neurotrophic Signaling Pathway Slow Alzheimer's Disease?" *International Journal of Molecular Sciences*, 2017.

[166] Gahee Bahn, Jong-Sung Park, Ui Jeong Yun, Yoon Jee Lee, Yuri Choi, Jin Su Park, Seung Hyun Baek, Bo Youn Choi, Yoon Suk Cho, Hark Kyun Kim, Jihoon Han, Jae Hoon Sul, Sang-Ha Baik, Jinhwan Lim, Nobunao Wakabayashi, Soo Han Bae, Jeung-Whan Han, Thiruma V. Arumugam, Mark P. Mattson and Dong-Gyu Jo. "NRF2/ARE Pathway Negatively Regulates BACE1 Expression and Ameliorates Cognitive Deficits in Mouse Alzheimer's Models." *Proceedings of the National Academy of Sciences of the U S A*, 2019.

[167] R. Kannan, J. F. Kuhlenkamp, E. Jeandidier, H. Trinh, M. Ookhtens and N. Kaplowitz. "Evidence for Carrier-Mediated Transport of Glutathione Across the Blood-Brain Barrier in the Rat." *The Journal of Clinical Investigation*, 1990.

[168] Jörg B. Schulz, Jörg Lindenau, Jan Seyfried and Johannes Dichgans. "Glutathione, Oxidative Stress and Neurodegeneration." *European Journal of Biochemistry*, 2000.

[169] Angélica Saraí Jiménez-Osorio, Susana González-Reyes and José Pedraza-Chaverri. "Natural Nrf2 Activators in Diabetes." *Clinica Chimica Acta*, 2015.

[170] Jamilah Abusarah, Houda Benabdoune, Qin Shi, Bertrand Lussier, Johanne Martel-Pelletier, Michel Malo, Julio C. Fernandes, Fátima Pereira de Souza, Hassan Fahmi and Mohamed Benderdour. "Elucidating the Role of Protandim and 6-Gingerol in Protection Against Osteoarthritis." *Journal of Cellular Biochemistry*, 2017.

[171] Brooks M. Hybertson, Bifeng Gao, Swapan K. Bose and Joe M. McCord. "Oxidative Stress in Health and Disease: The Therapeutic Potential of Nrf2 Activation." *Molecular Aspects of Medicine*, 2011.

[172] M. Flint Beal. "Coenzyme Q10 Administration and its Potential for Treatment of Neurodegenerative Diseases." *BioFactors*, 1999.

[173] Kazumasa Yamagishi, Ai Ikeda, Yuri Moriyama, Choy-Lye Chei, Hiroyuki Noda, Mitsumasa Umesawa, Renzhe Cui, Masanori Nagao, Akihiko Kitamura, Yorihiro Yamamoto, Takashi Asada, Hiroyasu Iso and CIRCS Investigators. "Serum Coenzyme Q10 and Risk of Disabling Dementia: The Circulatory Risk in Communities Study (CIRCS)." *Atherosclerosis*, 2014.

[174] Alexander Storch, Wolfgang H. Jost, Peter Vieregge, Jörg Spiegel, Wolfgang Greulich, Joachim Durner, Thomas Müller, Andreas Kupsch, Henning Henningsen, Wolfgang H. Oertel, Gerd Fuchs, Wilfried Kuhn, Petra Niklowitz, Rainer Koch, Birgit

Herting, Heinz Reichmann and German Coenzyme Q(10) Study Group. "Randomized, Double-Blind, Placebo-Controlled Trial on Symptomatic Effects of Coenzyme Q(10) in Parkinson Disease." *Archives of Neurology*, 2007.

[175] Andrew McGarry, Michael McDermott, Karl Kieburtz, Elisabeth A. de Blieck, Flint Beal, Karen Marder, Christopher Ross, Ira Shoulson, Peter Gilbert, William M. Mallonee, Mark Guttman, Joanne Wojcieszek, Rajeev Kumar, Mark S. LeDoux, Mary Jenkins, H. Diana Rosas, Martha Nance, Kevin Biglan, Peter Como, Richard M. Dubinsky, Kathleen M. Shannon, Padraig O'Suilleabhain 2, Kelvin Chou 2, Francis Walker 2, Wayne Martin 2, Vicki L Wheelock 2, Elizabeth McCusker, Joseph Jankovic, Carlos Singer, Juan Sanchez-Ramos, Burton Scott, Oksana Suchowersky, Stewart A. Factor, Donald S. Higgins, Jr., Eric Molho, Fredy Revilla, John N. Caviness, Joseph H. Friedman, Joel S. Perlmutter, Andrew Feigin, Karen Anderson, Ramon Rodriguez, Nikolaus R. McFarland, Russell L. Margolis, Eric S. Farbman, Lynn A. Raymond, Valerie Suski, Sandra Kostyk, Amy Colcher, Lauren Seeberger, Eric Epping, Sherali Esmail, Nancy Diaz, Wai Lun Alan Fung, Alan Diamond, Samuel Frank, Philip Hanna, Neal Hermanowicz, Leon S. Dure, Merit Cudkowicz and Huntington Study Group 2CARE Investigators and Coordinators. "A Randomized, Double-Blind, Placebo-Controlled Trial of Coenzyme Q10 in Huntington Disease." *Neurology*, 2017.

[176] Javier Frontiñán-Rubio, Francisco J. Sancho-Bielsa, Juan R. Peinado, Frank M. LaFerla, Lydia Giménez-Llort, Mario Durán-Prado and Francisco J. Alcain. "Sex-Dependent Co-Occurrence of Hypoxia and β-Amyloid Plaques in Hippocampus and Entorhinal Cortex is Reversed by Long-Term Treatment with Ubiquinol and Ascorbic Acid in the 3 × Tg-AD Mouse Model of Alzheimer's Disease." *Molecular and Cellular Neurosciences*, 2018.

[177] Farzad Salehpour, Fereshteh Farajdokht, Javad Mahmoudi, Marjan Erfani, Mehdi Farhoudi, Pouran Karimi, Seyed Hossein Rasta, Saeed Sadigh-Eteghad, Michael R. Hamblin and Albert Gjedde. "Photobiomodulation and Coenzyme Q10 Treatments

Attenuate Cognitive Impairment Associated with Model of Transient Global Brain Ischemia in Artificially Aged Mice." *Frontiers in Cellular Neuroscience*, 2019.

[178] Abhinav Sharma, Gregg C. Fonarow, Javed Butler, Justin A. Ezekowitz and G. Michael Felker. "Coenzyme Q10 and Heart Failure: A State-of-the-Art Review." *Circulation: Heart Failure*, 2016.

[179] Chen Xu, Junhua Zhang, Doina M. Mihai and Ilyas Washington. "Light-Harvesting Chlorophyll Pigments Enable Mammalian Mitochondria to Capture Photonic Energy and Produce ATP." *Journal of Cell Science*, 2014.

[180] M. R. Ven Murthy, Prabhakar K. Ranjekar, Charles Ramassamy and Manasi Deshpande. "Scientific Basis for the Use of Indian Ayurvedic Medicinal Plants in the Treatment of Neurodegenerative Disorders: Ashwagandha." *Central Nervous System Agents in Medicinal Chemistry*, 2010.

[181] Narendra Singh, Mohit Bhalla, Prashanti de Jager and Marilena Gilca. "An Overview on Ashwagandha: A Rasayana (Rejuvenator) of Ayurveda." *African Journal of Traditional, Complementary and Alternative Medicines*, 2011.

[182] Dnyanraj Choudhary, Sauvik Bhattacharyya and Sekhar Bose. "Efficacy and Safety of Ashwagandha (Withania somnifera (L.) Dunal) Root Extract in Improving Memory and Cognitive Functions." *Journal of Dietary Supplements*, 2017.

[183] Nawab John Dar and Muzamil Ahmad. "Neurodegenerative Diseases and Withania Somnifera (L.): An Update." *Journal of Ethnopharmacology*, 2020.

[184] Sultan Zahiruddin, Parakh Basist, Abida Parveen, Rabea Parveen, Washim Khan, Gaurav and Sayeed Ahmad. "Ashwagandha in Brain Disorders: A Review of Recent Developments." *Journal of Ethnopharmacology*, 2020.

[185] Chuenjid Kongkeaw, Piyameth Dilokthornsakul, Phurit Thanarangsarit, Nanteetip Limpeanchob and C. Norman Scholfield. "Meta-Analysis of Randomized Controlled Trials on Cognitive Effects of Bacopa Monnieri Extract." *Journal of Ethnopharmacology*, 2014.

[186] Ananya Sadhu, Prabhat Upadhyay, Aruna Agrawal, Kaliappan Ilango, Dipankar Karmakar, Gur Prit Inder Singh and Govind Prasad Dubey. "Management of Cognitive Determinants in Senile Dementia of Alzheimer's Type: Therapeutic Potential of a Novel Polyherbal Drug Product." *Clinical Drug Investigation*, 2014.

[187] Jintang Wang, Yuetao Song, Zheng Chen and Sean X. Leng. "Connection Between Systemic Inflammation and Neuroinflammation Underlies Neuroprotective Mechanism of Several Phytochemicals in Neurodegenerative Diseases." *Oxidative Medicine and Cellular Longevity*, 2018.

[188] Heather M. Wilkins and Russell H. Swerdlow. "Relationships Between Mitochondria and Neuroinflammation: Implications for Alzheimer's Disease." *Current Topics in Medicinal Chemistry*, 2016.

[189] Jintang Wang, Yuetao Song, Maolong Gao, Xujing Bai and Zheng Chen. "Neuroprotective Effect of Several Phytochemicals and Its Potential Application in the Prevention of Neurodegenerative Diseases." *Geriatrics*, 2016.

[190] Rita Moretti and Paola Caruso. "The Controversial Role of Homocysteine in Neurology: From Labs to Clinical Practice." *International Journal of Molecular Sciences*, 2019.

[191] Hassan Rasouli, Mohammad Hosein Farzaei and Reza Khodarahmi. "Polyphenols and Their Benefits: A Review." *International Journal of Food Properties*, 2017.

[192] Jintang Wang, Yuetao Song, Zheng Chen and Sean X. Leng. "Connection Between Systemic Inflammation and Neuroinflammation Underlies Neuroprotective Mechanism of

Several Phytochemicals in Neurodegenerative Diseases." *Oxidative Medicine and Cellular Longevity*, 2018.

[193] Syed-Badrul Syarifah-Noratiqah, Isa Naina-Mohamed, Mohamed S. Zulfarina and H. M. S. Qodriyah. "Natural Polyphenols in the Treatment of Alzheimer's Disease." *Current Drug Targets*, 2018.

[194] Thomas G. Balshaw, Theodoros M. Bampouras, Timothy J. Barry and S. Andy Sparks. "The Effect of Acute Taurine Ingestion on 3-km Running Performance in Trained Middle-Distance Runners." *Amino Acids*, 2013.

[195] Christine Perdan Curran and Cecile A. Marczinski. "Taurine, Caffeine, and Energy Drinks: Reviewing the Risks to the Adolescent Brain." *Birth Defects Research*, 2017.

[196] Gregory E. Bigford and Gianluca Del Rossi. "Supplemental Substances Derived from Foods as Adjunctive Therapeutic Agents for Treatment of Neurodegenerative Diseases and Disorders." *Advances in Nutrition*, 2014.

[197] Emiliano Albanese, Alan D. Dangour, Ricardo Uauy, Daisy Acosta, Mariella Guerra, Sara S. Gallardo Guerra, Yueqin Huang, K. S. Jacob, Juan Llibre de Rodriguez, Lisseth Hernandex Noriega, Aquiles Salas, Ana Luisa Sosa, Renata M Sousa, Joseph Williams, Cleusa P. Ferri and Martin J. Prince. "Dietary Fish and Meat Intake and Dementia in Latin America, China, and India: A 10/66 Dementia Research Group Population-Based Study." *The American Journal of Clinical Nutrition*, 2009.

[198] Paul Giem, W. Lawrence Beeson and Gary E. Fraser. "The Incidence of Dementia and Intake of Animal Products: Preliminary Findings From the Adventist Health Study." *Neuroepidemiology*, 1993.

[199] Alina Kepka, Agnieszka Ochocinska, Małgorzata Borzym-Kluczyk, Ewa Skorupa, Beata Stasiewicz-Jarocka, Sylwia Chojnowska and Napoleon Waszkiewicz. "Preventive Role of L-

Carnitine and Balanced Diet in Alzheimer's Disease." *Nutrients*, 2020.

[200] Steven T. DeKosky, Jeff D. Williamson, Annette L. Fitzpatrick, Richard A. Kronmal, Diane G. Ives, Judith A. Saxton, Oscar L. Lopez, Gregory Burke, Michelle C. Carlson, Linda P. Fried, Lewis H. Kuller, John A. Robbins, Russell P. Tracy, Nancy F. Woolard, Leslie Dunn, Beth E. Snitz, Richard L. Nahin, Curt D. Furberg and Ginkgo Evaluation of Memory (GEM) Study Investigators. "Ginkgo Biloba for Prevention of Dementia: A Randomized Controlled Trial." Published Correction Appears in *JAMA*, 2008.

[201] Thammanard Charemboon and Kankamol Jaisin. "Ginkgo Biloba for Prevention of Dementia: A Systematic Review and Meta-Analysis." *Journal of the Medical Association of Thailand*, 2015.

[202] Mengmeng Yang, Dan Dan Xu, Yan Zhang, Xinyou Liu, Robin Hoeven and William Chi Shing Cho. "A Systematic Review on Natural Medicines for the Prevention and Treatment of Alzheimer's Disease with Meta-Analyses of the Intervention Effect of Ginkgo." *The American Journal of Chinese Medicine*, 2014.

[203] Egemen Savaskan, Heiko Mueller, Robert Hoerr, Armin von Gunten and Serge Gauthier. "Treatment Effects of Ginkgo Biloba Extract EGb 761® on the Spectrum of Behavioral and Psychological Symptoms of Dementia: Meta-Analysis of Randomized Controlled Trials." *International Psychogeriatrics*, 2018.

[204] Serge Gauthier and Sandra Schlaefke. "Efficacy and Tolerability of Ginkgo Biloba Extract EGb 761® in Dementia: A Systematic Review and Meta-Analysis of Randomized Placebo-Controlled Trials." *Clinical Interventions in Aging*, 2014.

[205] Rainer Spiegel, Roger Kalla, Georgios Mantokoudis, Raphael Maire, Heiko Mueller, Robert Hoerr and Ralf Ihl. "Ginkgo Biloba Extract EGb 761® Alleviates Neurosensory Symptoms in Patients with Dementia: A Meta-Analysis of Treatment Effects on Tinnitus

and Dizziness in Randomized, Placebo-Controlled Trials." *Clinical Interventions in Aging*, 2018.

[206] Meng-Shan Tan, Jin-Tai Yu, Chen-Chen Tan, Hui-Fu Wang, Xiang-Fei Meng, Chong Wang, Teng Jiang, Xi-Chen Zhu and Lan Tan. "Efficacy and Adverse Effects of Ginkgo Biloba for Cognitive Impairment and Dementia: A Systematic Review and Meta-Analysis." *Journal of Alzheimer's Disease*, 2015.

[207] Ken Kihara, Hirohito M. Kondo and Jun I. Kawahara. "Differential Contributions of GABA Concentration in Frontal and Parietal Regions to Individual Differences in Attentional Blink." *The Journal of Neuroscience*, 2016.

[208] Anna Leonte, Lorenza S. Colzato, Laura Steenbergen, Bernhard Hommel and Elkan G. Akyürek. "Supplementation of Gamma-Aminobutyric Acid (GABA) Affects Temporal, But Not Spatial Visual Attention." *Brain and Cognition*, 2018.

[209] Evert Boonstra, Roy de Kleijn, Lorenza S. Colzato, Anneke Alkemade, Birte U. Forstmann, and Sander Nieuwenhuis. "Neurotransmitters as Food Supplements: The Effects of GABA on Brain and Behavior." *Frontiers in Psychology*, 2015.

[210] "HeartDisease and Homocysteine." WebMD, 2020. https://www.webmd.com/heart-disease/guide/homocysteine-risk#:~:text

[211] Arturo J. Martí-Carvajal, Ivan Solà, Dimitrios Lathyris and Mark Dayer. "Homocysteine-Lowering Interventions for Preventing Cardiovascular Events." *The Cochrane Database of Systemic Reviews*, 2017.

[212] David S. Wald, Anuradhani Kasturiratne and Mark Simmonds. "Serum Homocysteine and Dementia: Meta-Analysis of Eight Cohort Studies Including 8669 Participants." *Alzheimer's & Dementia*, 2011.

[213] Thorleif Etgen, Dirk Sander, Horst Bickel and Hans Förstl. "Mild Cognitive Impairment and Dementia: The Importance of Modifiable Risk Factors." *Deutsches Ärzteblatt International*, 2011.

[214] Liang Shen and Hong-Fang Ji. "Associations Between Homocysteine, Folic Acid, Vitamin B12 and Alzheimer's Disease: Insights from Meta-Analyses." *Journal of Alzheimer's Disease*, 2015.

[215] Yi Xie, Hongliang Feng, Sisi Peng, Jinsong Xiao and Junjian Zhang. "Association of Plasma Homocysteine, Vitamin B12 and Folate Levels with Cognitive Function in Parkinson's Disease: A Meta-Analysis." *Neuroscience Letters*, 2017.

[216] Anne Ws Rutjes, David A. Denton, Marcello Di Nisio, Lee-Yee Chong, Rajesh P. Abraham, Aalya S. Al-Assaf, John L. Anderson, Muzaffar A. Malik, Robin Wm Vernooij, Gabriel Martínez, Naji Tabet, Jenny McCleery. "Vitamin and Mineral Supplementation for Maintaining Cognitive Function in Cognitively Healthy People in Mid and Late Life." *The Cochrane Database of Systematic Reviews*, 2018.

[217] Andrew H. Ford and Osvaldo P. Almeida. "Effect of Homocysteine Lowering Treatment on Cognitive Function: A Systematic Review and Meta-Analysis of Randomized Controlled Trials." *Journal of Alzheimer's Disease*, 2012.

[218] Arturo J. Martí-Carvajal, Ivan Solà, Dimitrios Lathyris and Mark Dayer. "Homocysteine-Lowering Interventions for Preventing Cardiovascular Events." *The Cochrane Database of Systematic Reviews*, 2017.

[219] Caldwell B. Esselstyn, Jr. "Defining an Overdue Requiem for Palliative Cardiovascular Medicine." *American Journal of Lifestyle Medicine*, 2016.

[220] Michael F. Holick. "Vitamin D Deficiency." *The New England Journal of Medicine*, 2007.

[221] Michael F. Holick, Lois Y. Matsuoka and Jacobo Wortsman. "Age, Vitamin D, and Solar Ultraviolet." *The Lancet*, 1989.

[222] A. Pines. "Vitamin D and Health Issues--Questioned Benefits." *Climacteric*, 2014.

[223] Véréna Landel, Cédric Annweiler, Pascal Millet, Maria Morello and François Féron. "Vitamin D, Cognition and Alzheimer's Disease: The Therapeutic Benefit is in the D-Tails." *Journal of Alzheimer's Disease*, 2016.

[224] Ahmad Jayedi, Ali Rashidy-Pour and Sakineh Shab-Bidar. "Vitamin D Status and Risk of Dementia and Alzheimer's Disease: A Meta-Analysis of Dose-Response." *Nutritional Neuroscience*, 2019.

[225] Sadia Sultan, Uzma Taimuri, Shatha Abdulrzzaq Basnan, Waad Khalid Ai-Orabi, Afaf Awadallah, Fatimah Almowald and Amira Hazazi. "Low Vitamin D and Its Association with Cognitive Impairment and Dementia." *Journal of Aging Research*, 2020.

[226] Véréna Landel, Cédric Annweiler, Pascal Millet, Maria Morello and François Féron. "Vitamin D, Cognition and Alzheimer's Disease: The Therapeutic Benefit is in the D-Tails." *Journal of Alzheimer's Disease*, 2016.

[227] Edgar R. Miller 3rd, Roberto Pastor-Barriuso, Darshan Dalal, Rudolph A. Riemersma, Lawrence J. Appel and Eliseo Guallar. "Meta-Analysis: High-Dosage Vitamin E Supplementation May Increase All-Cause Mortality." *Annals of Internal Medicine*, 2005.

[228] Erin L. Abner, Frederick A. Schmitt, Marta S. Mendiondo, Jennifer L. Marcum and Richard J. Kryscio. "Vitamin E and All-Cause Mortality: A Meta-Analysis." *Current Aging Science*, 2011.

[229] Andrea J. Curtis, Michael Bullen, Loretta Piccenna and John J. McNeil. "Vitamin E Supplementation and Mortality in Healthy People: A Meta-Analysis of Randomized Controlled Trials." *Cardiovascular Drugs and Therapy*, 2014.

[230] Agnese Gugliandolo, Placido Bramanti and Emanuela Mazzon. "Role of Vitamin E in the Treatment of Alzheimer's Disease: Evidence from Animal Models." *International Journal of Molecular Science*, 2017.

[231] Mehrdad Jahanshahi, Emsehgol Nikmahzar and Ali Sayyahi. "Vitamin E Therapy Prevents the Accumulation of Congophilic Amyloid Plaques and Neurofibrillary Tangles in the Hippocampus in a Rat Model of Alzheimer's Disease." *Iran Journal of Basic Medical Science*, 2020.

[232] Declan Browne, Bernadette McGuinness, Jayne V. Woodside and Gareth J. McKay. "Vitamin E and Alzheimer's Disease: What Do We Know So Far?" *Clinical Interventions in Aging*, 2019.

[233] Richard J. Kryscio, Erin L. Abner, Allison Caban-Holt, Mark Lovell, Phyllis Goodman, Amy K. Darke, Monica Yee, John Crowley and Frederick A. Schmitt. "Association of Antioxidant Supplement Use and Dementia in the Prevention of Alzheimer's Disease by Vitamin E and Selenium Trial (PREADViSE)." *JAMA Neurology*, 2017.

[234] Nicolas Farina, David Llewellyn, Mokhtar Gad El Kareem Nasr Isaac and Naji Tabet. Vitamin E for Alzheimer's Dementia and Mild Cognitive Impairment." *The Cochrane Database of Systematic Reviews*, 2017.

[235] Dagfinn Aune, NaNa Keum, Edward Giovannucci, Lars T. Fadnes, Paolo Boffetta, Darren C. Greenwood, Serena Tonstad, Lars J. Vatten, Elio Riboli and Teresa Norat. "Dietary Intake and Blood Concentrations of Antioxidants and the Risk of Cardiovascular Disease, Total Cancer, and All-Cause Mortality: A Systematic Review and Dose-Response Meta-Analysis of Prospective Studies." *The American Journal of Clinical Nutrition*, 2018.

[236] Daniela Mastroiacovo, Catherine Kwik-Uribe, Davide Grassi, Stefano Necozione, Angelo Raffaele, Luana Pistacchio, Roberta

Righetti, Raffaella Bocale, Maria Carmela Lechiara, Carmine Marini, Claudio Ferri and Giovambattista Desideri. "Cocoa Flavanol Consumption Improves Cognitive Function, Blood Pressure Control, and Metabolic Profile in Elderly Subjects: The Cocoa, Cognition, and Aging (CoCoA) Study--A Randomized Controlled Trial." *The American Journal of Clinical Nutrition*, 2015.

[237] Richard P. Sloan, Melanie M. Wall, Lok-Kin Yeung, Tianshu Feng, Xinyang Feng, Frank Provenzano, Hagen Schroeter, Vincenzo Lauriola, Adam M. Brickman and Scott Small. "Insights Into the Role of Diet and Dietary Flavanols in Cognitive Aging: Results of a Randomized Controlled Trial." *Scientific Reports*, 2021.

[238] Sloan, Wall, Yeung, Feng, Feng, Provenzano, Schroeter, Lauriola, Brickman and Small. "Insights Into the Role of Diet and Dietary Flavanols in Cognitive Aging: Results of a Randomized Controlled Trial."

[239] Pauline Anderson. "Multivitamins, But Not Cocoa, Tied to Slowed Brain Aging." Medscape, 2021.

[240] Michael C. Craig, Pauline M. Maki and Declan G. M. Murphy. "The Women's Health Initiative Memory Study: Findings and Implications for Treatment." *The Lancet: Neurology*, 2005.

[241] Patricia Van Leer. "The Risk of Cardiovascular Disease, Fracture, Dementia, and Cancer After Long-Term Hormone Therapy in Perimenopausal and Postmenopausal Women." *American Family Physician*, 2018.

[242] Pauline M. Maki and Victor W. Henderson. "Hormone Therapy, Dementia, and Cognition: The Women's Health Initiative 10 Years On." *Climacteric*, 2012.

[243] Victor Henderson, Kelly Suzanne Benke, R. C. Green, L. A. Cupples, Lindsay Farrer and MIRAGE Study Group. "Postmenopausal Hormone Therapy and Alzheimer's Disease Risk:

Interaction with Age." *Journal of Neurology, Neurosurgery, and Psychiatry*, 2005.

[244] Rachel A. Whitmer, Charles P. Quesenberry, Jufen Zhou and Kristine Yaffe. "Timing of Hormone Therapy and Dementia: The Critical Window Theory Revisited." *Annals of Neurology*, 2011.

[245] Pauline M. Maki and Victor W. Henderson. "Hormone Therapy, Dementia, and Cognition: The Women's Health Initiative 10 Years On." *Climacteric*, 2012.

[246] Alzheimer, A. on peculiar cases of illness in later years. Z. fdg Neur U. Psych. 1911. https://doi.org/10.1007/BF02866241.

[247] Vincent Chin-Hung Chen, Shu-I Wu, Kuo-You Huang, Yao-Hsu Yang, Ting-Yu Kuo, Hsin-Yi Liang, Kuan-Lun Huang and Michael Gossop. "Herpes Zoster and Dementia: A Nationwide Population-Based Cohort Study." *The Journal of Clinical Psychiatry*, 2018.

[248] Ghulam M. Ashraf, Vadim V. Tarasov, Alfiya Makhmutova, Vladimir N. Chubarev, Marco Avila-Rodriguez, Sergey O. Bachurin and Gjumrakch Aliev. "The Possibility of an Infectious Etiology of Alzheimer Disease." *Molecular Neurobiology*, 2019.

[249] James Stefaniak and John O'Brien. "Imaging of Neuroinflammation in Dementia: A Review." *Journal of Neurology, Neurosurgery, and Psychiatry*, 2016.

[250] Nian-Sheng Tzeng, Chi-Hsiang Chung, Fu-Huang Lin, Chien-Ping Chiang, Chin-Bin Yeh, San-Yuan Huang, Ru-Band Lu, Hsin-An Chang, Yu-Chen Kao, Hui-Wen Yeh, Wei-Shan Chiang, Yu-Ching Chou, Chang-Huei Tsao, Yung-Fu Wu and Wu-Chien Chien. "Anti-Herpetic Medications and Reduced Risk of Dementia in Patients with Herpes Simplex Virus Infections-a Nationwide, Population-Based Cohort Study in Taiwan." *Neurotherapeutics*, 2018.

[251] Avindra Nath. "Association of Herpes Viral Infections, Antiherpetic Therapy, and Dementia: Real or Alternative Fact?" *Neurotherapeutics*, 2018.

[252] Avindra Nath. "Herpes Viruses, Alzheimer's Disease, and Related Dementias: Unifying or Confusing Hypothesis?" *Neurotherapeutics*, 2019.

[253] M. Torniainen-Holm, J. Suvisaari, M. Lindgren, T. Härkänen, F. Dickerson and R. H. Yolken. "The Lack of Association Between Herpes Simplex Virus 1 or Toxoplasma Gondii Infection and Cognitive Decline in the General Population: An 11-Year Follow-Up Study." *Brain, Behavior, and Immunity*, 2019.

[254] Ruth F. Itzhaki. "Herpes and Alzheimer's Disease: Subversion in the Central Nervous System and How It Might Be Halted." *Journal of Alzheimer's Disease*, 2016.

[255] Ruth Alonso, Diana Pisa, Ana Isabel Marina, Esperanza Morato, Alberto Rábano and Luis Carrasco. "Fungal Infection in Patients with Alzheimer's Disease." *Journal of Alzheimer's Disease*, 2014.

[256] Diana Pisa, Ruth Alonso, Ana M. Fernández-Fernández, Alberto Rábano and Luis Carrasco. "Polymicrobial Infections in Brain Tissue from Alzheimer's Disease Patients." *Scientific Reports*, 2017.

[257] Ruth Alonso, Diana Pisa, Ana M. Fernández-Fernández and Luis Carrasco. "Infection of Fungi and Bacteria in Brain Tissue from Elderly Persons and Patients with Alzheimer's Disease." *Frontiers in Aging Neuroscience*, 2018.

[258] Róisín M. McManus and Michael T. Heneka. "Role of Neuroinflammation in Neurodegeneration: New Insights." *Alzheimer's Research & Therapy*, 2017.

[259] Róisín M. McManus, Kingston H. G. Mills and Marina A. Lynch. "T Cells-Protective or Pathogenic in Alzheimer's Disease?" *Journal of Neuroimmune Pharmacology*, 2015.

[260] Ruth Alonso, Diana Pisa, Ana M. Fernández-Fernández and Luis Carrasco. "Infection of Fungi and Bacteria in Brain Tissue from Elderly Persons and Patients with Alzheimer's Disease." *Frontiers in Aging Neuroscience*, 2018.

About the Author

Cliff Arceneaux is a graduate of Wake Forest University's School of Medicine, and has been working full time as a Physician Associate since 2006. His work has taken him from busy nights in the ER with cardiology to working in prison infirmaries. For the past 10 years, he has been working in Geriatrics, taking care of patients in the office, in facilities or in their homes. Working with folks in the 80s, 90s and beyond is a most satisfying challenge. Getting patients to buy into making lifestyle choices to replace their medications can be tricky, but very rewarding. Cliff always counts it as a good day when an 85-year-old patient shows up with stronger legs and a sturdier mind simply by trading in pills for broccoli and a daily walk.

Printed in Great Britain
by Amazon

47286296R00099